WITHDRAWN

Methodology in Medical Genetics

To my teachers
R.P.
and
V.A.M.
with much respect

Methodology in Medical Genetics

An Introduction to Statistical Methods

Alan E. H. Emery
M.D., Ph.D., D.Sc., F.R.C.P.(E.), M.F.C.M., F.R.S.(E.)
Professor of Human Genetics,
University of Edinburgh

CHURCHILL LIVINGSTONE
Edinburgh London and New York 1976

CHURCHILL LIVINGSTONE

Medical Division of Longman Group Limited

Distributed in the United States of America by
Longman Inc., 19 West 44th Street, New York, N.Y. 10036
and by associated companies, branches and representatives
throughout the world.

First published 1976

ISBN 0 443 01438 8

Library of Congress Cataloging in Publication Data

Emery, Alan E. H.
    Methodology in medical genetics.

    Bibliography: p.
    Includes index.
    1. Medical genetics—Statistical methods.
I. Title. [DNLM: 1. Biometry. 2. Genetics, Human. QH431 E53m]
RB155.E52   616′.042   76-8946

Printed in Great Britain

Preface

This is not intended to be a textbook but rather a practical guide to simple statistical methods of use to those with a particular interest in Medical Genetics. The emphasis throughout is on the solution of practical, rather than theoretical, problems and particularly on problems of medical importance.

It is assumed that the reader has some knowledge of human genetics and an acquaintance with very simple statistics, but a level of mathematical sophistication no greater than simple algebra is required.

An effort has been made to make the book more or less self-contained with sufficient information, in the form of worked examples and reference tables, to enable the reader to apply the methods to his or her own data. It is hoped that the book will at least encourage, and perhaps help, those who would like to attempt to analyse their own data themselves armed with no more than log tables or a hand calculator.

A.E.H.E.

Edinburgh/Ibiza,
1976

Acknowledgements

Any faults in this little book are clearly mine. There would have been many more except for colleagues and friends who have so generously given up their time to read and advise me on particular chapters and sections. In particular I should like to thank Dr A. M. Davie, F.R.S.(E.), Professor D. S. Falconer, F.R.S., Mr W. Lutz, Dr R. Morton, Dr Ruth Sanger, F.R.S., Dr J. Shields and Professor C. A. B. Smith. I am especially grateful to Professor W. J. Schull and Dr Charles Smith who read the entire script and made many helpful suggestions and Dr Susan Holloway who graciously accepted the onerous task of checking my calculations.

I am most grateful to Mr J. E. Pizer for preparing the illustrations and to the following authors and publishers for permission to use various tables and figures: Table 4.3 (W. W. Norton, Inc., New York), Table 4.5 (Professor C. C. Li and McGraw-Hill Inc., New York), Table 4.6 (Professor C. C. Li and Dr N. Mantel and the editor and publishers of the *American Journal of Human Genetics*), Figure 5.2 (Dr Charles Smith and the editor and publishers of the *Annals of Human Genetics (London)*), Figure 7.3 (Dr R. E. Gaines and Dr R. C. Elston and the editor and publishers of the *American Journal of Human Genetics*), Table 10.2 (Professor C. A. B. Smith and the editor and publishers of the *Annals of Human Genetics (London)*), Table 11.3 (Dr D. Hewitt and the editor and publishers of the *British Journal of Preventive and Social Medicine*), Appendices 1, 2 and 3 (Professor N. T. J. Bailey and the English Universities Press), Appendix 4 (Dr R. R. Sokal and Dr F. J. Rohlf and Freeman Inc., San Francisco), Appendix 5 (Professor D. S. Falconer, F.R.S. and the editor and publishers of the *Annals of Human Genetics (London)*) and Appendix 6 (Professor C. A. B. Smith).

Finally this book would have been quite impossible without the assistance of my wife Rosalind and my secretary, Miss Margaret Fairbairn, and of course the criticisms of my students for whom this book was intended in the first place.

Contents

1. Introduction

In the last decade or so, developments in human biochemical genetics and cytogenetics have tended to eclipse quantitative methods in Medical Genetics. These methods, however, will always provide the basis for much research in the subject. Admittedly some have little practical value, as for example studies of genetic drift and effective population size, assortative mating and inbreeding, gene flow and racial admixture, and natural selection, but clearly the study and measurement of such phenomena are essential for any understanding and appreciation of man's evolution. In other areas there is potential practical value but this has not yet been exploited. This is true of gene mapping, though even here the recent demonstration that secretor status and myotonic dystrophy are linked has already proved valuable in the antenatal diagnosis of this disorder in certain families. It is only a matter of time before genetic linkage studies become widely applied to problems in genetic counselling and antenatal diagnosis.

Several of these statistical methods are particularly valuable in helping to elucidate the role of environmental factors in congenital malformations of unknown aetiology. Particularly useful in this regard are the techniques for recognizing and measuring changes in disease frequency and cyclical trends, and for estimating parental age and birth order effects.

The study of disease associations has taken a new lease of life with the recent discovery of strong associations with certain HLA types which may well throw light on the aetiology of those disorders with which they are associated, and though interest in twin studies has somewhat declined in recent years much valuable information concerning the nature versus nurture controversy can still be gained from such studies, particularly in the realm of psychiatric disorders.

Yet other techniques, either directly or indirectly, have yielded information of value in risk prediction for genetic counselling. The estimation of heritability is most valuable as a measure of genetic determination but such information can also be used to predict risks to relatives, and segregation analysis can help establish the mode of inheritance which is obviously important for genetic counselling. Methods for estimating recurrence risks, often employing statistical tools such as Bayes' theorem, have become increasingly important in recent years as the need for genetic counselling has become more widely accepted.

Some of these methods, however, are complicated and have occupied the attention of some of the best intellects in Human Genetics. For this reason the non-mathematically minded are sometimes discouraged. This book is specially written for those with a level of mathematical sophistication no greater than simple algebra. This of course means that rarely will the derivation and proof of an equation or relationship be given but in all such cases reference is made to where this information can be found. The reader, however, is assumed to have some knowledge of basic genetics and simple statistical methods and so be acquainted with such terms as standard error, statistical significance, correlation coefficient and chi square (χ^2).

The book is intended to be a simple straightforward *practical* guide to methods for analysing human genetic data. Each method is illustrated with worked examples from real data, either published or unpublished, and tables and graphs are included to help the reader with the calculations. The methods described are essentially those which can be applied by the individual investigator armed with no more than log tables or a desk calculator. Some refined methods, usually requiring a computer for analysis, have therefore been considered beyond the scope of this book. For example, the calculation of the coefficient of inbreeding from marriage distances and computer methods for discriminating between different modes of inheritance. One further point: particular data have been chosen because they illustrate a method of calculation and not because they necessarily (though they often do) represent the best available data on the subject. Since this is more a work book than a text book no serious attempt has been made to assess critically the results of such studies. However the problems and limitations of the various methods are emphasized and discussed, and references are given to original reports so that the interested reader may find more detailed treatment of a particular statistical method. The principal danger is the uncritical application of the methods described. If in doubt the reader should therefore always consult the original reference or an experienced colleague, which will be necessary, in any event, if the data warrant more complex analysis than is covered by this introduction, the aim of which was to deal only with simple basic methods.

It is hoped that the book is more or less self-contained with sufficient information to enable the reader to apply the methods to his or her own data, or at least help the reader to understand and perhaps appreciate more fully the studies of others.

2. Hardy-Weinberg Equilibrium and the Estimation of Gene Frequencies

Hardy-Weinberg equilibrium

Proposed by an English mathematician, G. H. Hardy, and a German physician, W. Weinberg, in 1908, the so-called Hardy-Weinberg principle can be expressed as follows. In a large, randomly mating (= panmixis) population, in which there is no migration, or selection against a particular genotype and the mutation rate remains constant, the proportions of the various genotypes will remain unchanged from one generation to another. An understanding of this principle is essential for much that will follow.

Consider two alleles 'A' and 'a' such that the proportion of 'A' genes is 'p' and the proportion of 'a' genes is 'q', then $p + q = 1$. *Throughout 'q' will be used to denote the frequency of the recessive allele.* Now with random mating the frequencies of the various genotypes will be:

Male gametes

		A (p)	a (q)
Female gametes	$A(p)$	AA (p^2)	Aa (pq)
	$a(q)$	Aa (pq)	aa (q^2)

Thus the frequencies of the various offspring from such matings are $p^2(AA)$, $2pq(Aa)$ and $q^2(aa)$, that is the terms of the expansion $(p + q)^2$.

If these progeny now mate with each other the frequencies of the various *matings* can be represented as:

Genotype frequency of male parent

		AA (p^2)	Aa $(2pq)$	aa (q^2)
Genotype frequency of female parent	AA (p^2)	p^4	$2p^3q$	p^2q^2
	Aa $(2pq)$	$2p^3q$	$4p^2q^2$	$2pq^3$
	aa (q^2)	p^2q^2	$2pq^3$	q^4

Thus, for example, the frequency of matings between persons with the genotypes 'aa' and 'Aa' is $2pq^3 + 2pq^3$ or $4pq^3$. The frequencies of the various *offspring* from these matings can be represented as:

Mating type	Frequency	Frequency of offspring		
		AA	Aa	aa
$AA \times AA$	p^4	p^4	—	—
$AA \times Aa$	$4p^3q$	$2p^3q$	$2p^3q$	—
$Aa \times Aa$	$4p^2q^2$	p^2q^2	$2p^2q^2$	p^2q^2
$AA \times aa$	$2p^2q^2$	—	$2p^2q^2$	—
$Aa \times aa$	$4pq^3$	—	$2pq^3$	$2pq^3$
$aa \times aa$	q^4	—	—	q^4

Total

$$
\begin{aligned}
&= p^2(p^2 + 2pq + q^2) + 2pq(p^2 + 2pq + q^2) + q^2(p^2 + 2pq + q^2) \\
&= \quad p^2(p + q)^2 \qquad + 2pq(p + q)^2 \qquad + q^2(p + q)^2 \\
&= \qquad\quad p^2 \qquad\quad + 2pq \qquad\qquad + q^2 \\
&= \quad (p + q)^2
\end{aligned}
$$

The *proportions* of the various genotypes remain the same in the second generation as in the first generation.

Estimation of autosomal gene frequencies

The method of estimation depends upon whether or not the heterozygote is recognizable.

Heterozygote is not recognizable
In this case there is complete dominance and therefore the heterozygote is not recognizable. Assuming that the genotypes are in equilibrium, then the gene frequencies can be estimated if the frequency of the rare homozygote is known. Thus in alkaptonuria (a recessive disorder) which affects about one child in every million:

$$q^2 = \frac{1}{1\ 000\ 000}$$

therefore
$$q = \frac{1}{1000}$$

but
$$p + q = 1$$

therefore
$$p \simeq 1$$

and the frequency of heterozygous carriers is $2pq$ or $1/500$.

The standard error of the estimation of 'q' (when the estimate of 'q' is based upon the frequency of homozygotes q^2) is $[(1 - q^2)/4N]^{\frac{1}{2}}$ where N is the number of individuals in the sample. Thus Pearn (1973) ascertained 9 cases of Werdnig-Hoffmann disease (a recessive disorder) in a total of 231 370 births in the North-East of England.

Therefore
$$q^2 = \frac{9}{231\ 370}$$

$$= 0{\cdot}000039$$

and
$$q = \sqrt{0{\cdot}000039}$$

$$= 0{\cdot}00624$$

and
$$\text{s.e.} = \sqrt{\frac{1 - 0{\cdot}000039}{(4)(231\ 370)}}$$

$$= 0{\cdot}00104$$

The 95 per cent confidence limits will therefore be

$$\text{mean} \pm 1{\cdot}96 \times \text{s.e.}$$

$$= 0{\cdot}00624 \pm 1{\cdot}96\ (0{\cdot}00104)$$

$$= 0{\cdot}00420 \text{ to } 0{\cdot}00828$$

Heterozygote is recognizable

If a characteristic is suspected of being determined by two co-dominant alleles, the heterozygote therefore being recognizable, the frequencies of the two genes can be estimated in the following way. For example in one study (Kellermann, Luyten-Kellermann and Shaw, 1973) the extent of induction of aryl hydrocarbon hydroxylase in human lymphocytes showed a trimodal distribution in the population and it was suggested that the three phenotypes represented the action of two alleles (A and B). Out of a total of 161 individuals investigated the phenotypic frequencies were:

$$\text{low inducibility} = 86\ (AA)$$

$$\text{intermediate inducibility} = 59\ (AB)$$

$$\text{high inducibility} = 16\ (BB)$$

$$\text{Therefore } A \text{ gene frequency} = \frac{86}{161} + \frac{1}{2}\left(\frac{59}{161}\right)$$

$$= 0{\cdot}717$$

$$\text{and } B \text{ gene frequency} = 1 - 0{\cdot}717$$

$$= 0{\cdot}283$$

Therefore the *expected* phenotype frequencies are:

$$AA = 161 \, (0 \cdot 717) \, (0 \cdot 717) \quad = 82 \cdot 8$$
$$AB = 161 \, (2) \, (0 \cdot 717) \, (0 \cdot 283) = 65 \cdot 3$$
$$BB = 161 \, (0 \cdot 283) \, (0 \cdot 283) \quad = 12 \cdot 9$$

To determine if the observed (O) and expected (E) results differ significantly we calculate the value of chi^2 (χ^2) which is equal to the square of the difference between O and E divided by E summed (represented by Greek letter sigma Σ) for all groups.

Thus:
$$\chi^2 = \Sigma \frac{(O - E)^2}{E}$$
$$= \frac{(3 \cdot 2)^2}{82 \cdot 8} + \frac{(6 \cdot 3)^2}{65 \cdot 3} + \frac{(3 \cdot 1)^2}{12 \cdot 9}$$
$$= 1 \cdot 48$$

We next determine the *number of degrees of freedom* (D.F.). In this sort of test—referred to as a 'goodness of fit' test—the number of degrees of freedom

$$= \text{(no. of classes)} - \text{(no. of estimated parameters)} - 1$$

In the above example there are three classes and there was one estimated parameter, namely the gene frequency, upon which the expected values were calculated. Therefore there is *one* degree of freedom. (The reader is referred to one of the standard text books of statistics for a discussion of the number of degrees of freedom in various statistical calculations.) With one degree of freedom, to be significant ($P < 0 \cdot 05$) the value of χ^2 would have to be greater than $3 \cdot 84$ (Appendix 2, p. 132). In fact the value of χ^2 is only $1 \cdot 48$ and therefore there is no significant difference between the observed and expected numbers of low, intermediate and high inducers if it is assumed that these phenotypes result from the operation of two codominant alleles.

Determination of the expected frequencies of various matings and the phenotypes of their offspring

Autosomal disorders

If it is considered that a certain characteristic could be due to the operation of two alleles, it is possible to determine the expected frequencies of the various types of matings, and the frequencies of the various types of offspring from these matings and to compare these findings with those observed.

For example, Evans, Manley and McKusick (1960) showed that it is possible to divide individuals into two classes according to their ability to metabolize the drug Isoniazid. These are referred to as 'rapid' and 'slow' inactivators. In order to determine if the slow inactivator phenotype represents the homozygous recessive genotype, Professor Price Evans and colleagues compared the observed and expected mating frequencies and their offspring. Out of a total of 291 individuals investigated the phenotype frequencies were:

$$\text{slow inactivators} = 152$$

$$\text{rapid inactivators} = 139$$

If *slow* inactivation represents the homozygous expression of an autosomal recessive gene (i.e. I_rI_r).

Then
$$I_rI_r(q^2) = \frac{152}{291}$$
$$= 0 \cdot 5223$$

therefore
$$I_r(q) = \sqrt{0 \cdot 5223}$$
$$= 0 \cdot 7227$$

and
$$I_R(p) = 1 - 0 \cdot 7227$$
$$= 0 \cdot 2773$$

Assuming random mating the number of expected mating types can then be calculated and compared with the observed numbers (Table 2.1).

Table 2.1 Numbers of observed matings compared with those expected if slow inactivation of isoniazid represents the homozygous expression of an autosomal recessive gene (Evans *et al.*, 1960)

Phenotypic matings	Genotypic matings	Expected frequency of matings		Expected occurrence in 53 matings	Observed occurrence
$S \times S$	$I_rI_r \times I_rI_r$	q^4	$0 \cdot 2728$	$14 \cdot 46$	16
$R \times S$	$I_RI_R \times I_rI_r$ $I_RI_r \times I_rI_r$	$2p^2q^2$ $4pq^3$	$\left.\begin{array}{c}0 \cdot 0803 \\ 0 \cdot 4187\end{array}\right\}\, 0 \cdot 4990$	$26 \cdot 45$	24
$R \times R$	$I_RI_R \times I_RI_R$ $I_RI_R \times I_RI_r$ $I_RI_r \times I_RI_r$	p^4 $4p^3q$ $4p^2q^2$	$\left.\begin{array}{c}0 \cdot 0059 \\ 0 \cdot 0616 \\ 0 \cdot 1606\end{array}\right\}\, 0 \cdot 2281$	$12 \cdot 09$	13

The observed and expected numbers of the different mating types can then be compared in the usual manner (Table 2.2).

Table 2.2 Comparison of the observed and expected numbers of matings in Table 2.1.

Mating	Observed	Expected	$(O - E)^2$	$\dfrac{(O - E)^2}{E}$
$S \times S$	16	14·46	2·372	0·164
$R \times S$	24	26·45	6·003	0·227
$R \times R$	13	12·09	0·828	0·0685
				$\chi^2 = \overline{0{\cdot}4595}$
				(D.F. = 1)

The value of χ^2 is 0·4595 which is not significant (Appendix 2, p. 132). Therefore the observed numbers of different mating types do not differ significantly from the expected numbers when it is assumed that slow inactivation represents the homozygous recessive genotype.

A further test of this hypothesis is to compare the expected with the observed numbers of children of each phenotype which result from various matings. Thus in matings between rapid and slow inactivators, assuming slow inactivation represents the homozygous recessive genotype, the expected proportion of slow inactivators $(I_r I_r)$ offspring is $2pq^3$ (p. 4), and the proportion among offspring resulting from this particular mating is:

$$\frac{2pq^3}{2pq^3 + 2p^2q^2 + 2pq^3}$$

$$= \frac{q}{p + 2q}$$

$$= \frac{0{\cdot}7227}{0{\cdot}2773 + 1{\cdot}4454}$$

$$= 0{\cdot}4195$$

Therefore the expected *number* of slow inactivator offspring among 70 offspring of matings between rapid and slow inactivators is

Table 2.3 Expected numbers of children of each isoniazid inactivator phenotype compared with those observed (Evans *et al.*, 1960)

Phenotypic matings	No. of matings	No. of children	Rapid E	Rapid O	Slow E	Slow O	χ^2	D.F.
$S \times S$	16	51	0	0	51	51	—	—
$R \times S$	24	70	40·62	42	29·36	28	0·110	1
$R \times R$	13	38	31·30	31	6·68	7	0·018	1
	53	159		73		86	0·128	2

No. of children of each phenotype

(70) (0·4195) or 29·36. Similarly the expected number of children of slow and rapid inactivator phenotype among the offspring of other matings can be determined (Table 2.3).

Since there is no significant difference between the observed and expected numbers, the data fit the hypothesis that slow inactivator phenotype represents the genetically homozygous recessive individual.

X-linked disorders

In an X-linked disorder the frequency of the mutant allele ('q') is equal to the incidence of the disorder among males. The frequencies of the various types of matings and the proportions of the various types of offspring from these matings can be represented as:

Mating type			Proportion among offspring of a given sex				
			Males		Females		
Male	Female	Frequency	a	A	aa	Aa	AA
a	AA	p^2q	—	1	—	1	—
a	Aa	$2pq^2$	$\frac{1}{2}$	$\frac{1}{2}$	$\frac{1}{2}$	$\frac{1}{2}$	—
a	aa	q^3	1	—	1	—	—
A	AA	p^3	—	1	—	—	1
A	Aa	$2p^2q$	$\frac{1}{2}$	$\frac{1}{2}$	—	$\frac{1}{2}$	$\frac{1}{2}$
A	aa	pq^2	1	—	—	1	—

As in the above example (p. 7), knowing 'q' it is possible to calculate:

1. The expected frequencies of various matings and compare these with the observed frequencies.

2. The expected frequencies of different types of offspring from various matings and compare these with the observed frequencies.

Estimation of multiple allele frequencies

When there are three alleles but only certain phenotypes can be recognized, gene frequencies have to be determined indirectly. For example, in the case of the ABO blood groups if the frequency of individuals with blood group O (OO) is represented as ($\bar{O}$), with blood group A (AA and AO) as ($\bar{A}$) and with blood group B (BB and BO) as ($\bar{B}$) then by simple algebra it can be shown that the gene frequencies are respectively:

$$I^A = \sqrt{(\bar{O}) + (\bar{A})} - \sqrt{(\bar{O})}$$

or

$$I^B = \frac{1 - \sqrt{\overline{(\overline{O})} + (\overline{\overline{B}})}}{\sqrt{(\overline{\overline{O}}) + (\overline{\overline{B}})} - \sqrt{(\overline{\overline{O}})}}$$

or

$$I^O = \frac{1 - \sqrt{(\overline{\overline{O}}) + (\overline{\overline{A}})}}{\sqrt{(\overline{\overline{O}})}}$$

When calculated in this way the sum of all the gene frequencies may not be equal to 1·00. There will be a deviation from unity referred to as 'D', where

$$D = \sqrt{(\overline{\overline{O}}) + (\overline{\overline{A}})} + \sqrt{(\overline{\overline{O}}) + (\overline{\overline{B}})} - \sqrt{\overline{\overline{O}}} - 1$$

An improved estimate of the gene frequencies can be obtained in the following way:

$$I^O = (1 + D/2)(\sqrt{(\overline{\overline{O}})} + D/2)$$
$$I^A = (1 + D/2)(1 - \sqrt{(\overline{\overline{O}}) + (\overline{\overline{B}})})$$
$$I^B = (1 + D/2)(1 - \sqrt{(\overline{\overline{O}}) + (\overline{\overline{A}})})$$

This and other methods of estimating blood group gene frequencies are clearly described in Race and Sanger (1975) and Levitan and Montagu (1971). ABO blood group gene frequencies in the United Kingdom are given in Table 2.4.

Table 2.4 Blood group gene frequencies in the United Kingdom (data selected from Mourant et al., 1958)

	A	B	O
England	0·252	0·050	0·698
Scotland	0·210	0·071	0·719
Wales	0·244	0·064	0·692
Northern Ireland	0·210	0·069	0·721
Overall	0·257	0·060	0·683

3. Estimation of Factors Affecting the Genetic Structure of Populations

We have seen that according to the Hardy-Weinberg principle it is assumed that the various genotypes in a population are in equilibrium, and their proportions therefore remain constant from one generation to another. However, this is only true in large populations with no *genetic drift,* and where there is random mating (panmixis) with no significant *assortative mating* or *inbreeding,* no *gene flow* from migration or racial admixture, no *selection* against a particular genotype and a constant rate of *mutation.* We shall now discuss how each of these factors can be estimated in a given population.

Genetic drift

In large populations random variations in the number of children produced by individuals with different genotypes has no significant effect on gene frequencies but this is not so in small populations ('*demes*' or '*isolates*') where such variations may have a considerable effect on gene frequencies (Sewall Wright effect). If only a few people carry a particular gene, if such individuals do not have children or they have children but by chance do not transmit this gene to their offspring, then, barring a fresh mutation, the gene in question will completely disappear from the population (Fig. 3.1) and is said to have been '*extinguished*' (gene frequency zero) and its allele to have become '*fixed*' (gene frequency 1·0). The amount of random genetic drift depends on the size of the population being greatest in small populations where oscillations in gene frequencies from one generation to another may be considerable.

Genetic drift is therefore a function of population size although not of *total* population size but rather the numbers of adults of breeding age and their ability to have offspring to contribute to the gene pool of the next generation. This is referred to as the *effective size* of the population or 'N_e'. Significant genetic drift is likely to occur in a given population whenever:

$$\mu, s \text{ or } m < 1/2N_e$$

where $\qquad\quad \mu = \text{mutation rate}$

$\qquad\qquad\quad s = \text{coefficient of selection}$

$\qquad\qquad\quad m = \text{migration rate}$

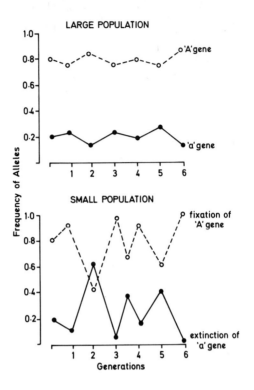

Fig. 3.1 The effects of genetic drift on gene frequencies in large and small populations (diagrammatic).

If the mutation rate is of the order of 10^{-6}, and if selection and migration are extremely low, then random genetic drift, can still be important in populations of an effective size of up to 250 000 (Wright, 1948).

In a small population, in the absence of mutation, selection or migration, the percentage of loci which will become fixed or eliminated in each generation is $100/2N_e$. Thus in a religious isolate in Pennsylvania, the so-called Old Order 'Dunker' (Old German Baptist) brethren, the community consisted of 298 individuals and the effective size of the population was estimated to be about 90 individuals (Glass et al., 1952). Therefore the percentage of loci which might be expected to become fixed or eliminated per generation in this community is 100/180 or 0·55 per cent, not an inconsiderable number of loci considering the possible size of the human genome.

Estimation of effective population size

Various equations have been developed in order to predict the effective size of the population under a variety of conditions which may exist in nature (Kimura and Crow, 1963). If the numbers of male (N_M) and female (N_F) parents are not equal then approximately:

$$N_e = \frac{4N_M N_F}{N_M + N_F}$$

Thus if in a particular population there were 50 males and 200 females of reproductive age, then:

$$N_e = \frac{4(50)(200)}{50 + 200}$$

$$= 160$$

Thus the effective size of the population is only 160 instead of 250. This could have been a significant factor in primitive societies in which polygyny (or polyandry) was practised.

For X-linked genes the effective size of the population is:

$$N_e = \frac{9N_M N_F}{4N_M + 2N_F}$$

Taking into account variation in number of offspring, and providing the population is fairly stable in size, then:

$$N_e = \frac{4N - 2}{V_o + 2}$$

where N = number of individuals of reproductive age
(say 15 to 45 years)

V_o = variance in number of offspring
(ideally those surviving to reproduction)

If necessary this can be computed independently for male and female parents, and separate estimates for the effective size of the population obtained for the two sexes.

Effective population size and gene frequencies
The variance in gene frequency is:

$$V_q = \frac{pq}{2N_e}$$

and therefore the expected (standard) deviation in one generation due to chance sampling is $\sqrt{V_q}$. Thus in the Cashinahua Indians, a genetic isolate in Peru, there were 206 individuals in 1966 of whom 87 were of reproductive age and the variance in offspring was 3·1 (Johnston *et al.*, 1969).

Therefore:

$$N_e = \frac{4(87) - 2}{3 \cdot 1 + 2}$$

$$= 68$$

Now the gene frequency of the Kidd blood group allele Jk^a was $0 \cdot 53$ (Johnston *et al.*, 1968) therefore:

$$\sqrt{V_q} = \sqrt{\frac{(0 \cdot 53)(0 \cdot 47)}{2(68)}}$$

$$= 0 \cdot 04$$

The 95 per cent confidence limits for the gene frequency in the next generation will therefore be $0 \cdot 53 \pm (1 \cdot 96)(0 \cdot 04)$ or $0 \cdot 45$ to $0 \cdot 61$ due to chance alone. After this, genetic drift would occur again in either direction the amount being a function of the new values of Jk^a and N_e. An interesting discussion of the genetic structure of an isolated primitive population is provided by Salzano, Neel and Maybury-Lewis (1967) in the case of the Xavante Indians of Brazil.

It should be noted that genetic drift would be particularly important in the spread of neutral genes. This has been referred to as non-Darwinian evolution in contrast to classical Darwinian evolution in which natural selection plays the major role (Thoday, 1975).

Assortative mating

The Hardy-Weinberg equilibrium only holds true if there is random mating (panmixis). *Assortative mating* and *inbreeding* disturb the equilibrium and result in an increase in the proportion of homozygotes and a decrease in the proportion of heterozygotes.

Assortative mating is usually concerned with resemblance between phenotypic traits such as height, intelligence, skin colouring and general physiognomy which have a multifactorial basis. In order to estimate the contribution of assortative mating to the total variance of a particular trait it is necessary to compute the following (Burt and Howard, 1956; Cavalli-Sforza and Bodmer, 1971):

$$C_1 C_2 = \frac{2r_{P/O}}{1 + r_{SP}}$$

$$\hat{A} = r_{SP}(C_1 C_2)$$

$$C_1 = 4r_{S/S} - C_1 C_2(1 + 2\hat{A})$$

where the correlation between spouses is 'r_{SP}', between parent and offspring is '$r_{P/O}$' and between sibs is '$r_{S/S}$'. The derivation of these formulae is given by Burt and Howard (1956).

The total variance of a trait is made up of environmental and genetic factors and (ignoring epistatic effects) the latter is due to the effects of dominant and additive genes (Falconer, 1960). These various components of the total variance can be calculated thus:

1. *Environmental* $\hspace{5cm} = 1 - C_1$

2. *Genetic*
   (a) Non-additive (due to dominance) $= C_1 - C_1 C_2$
   (b) Additive:
   expected under random mating $\hspace{0.5cm} = C_1 C_2 (1 - \hat{A})$
   due to assortative mating $\hspace{1.2cm} = C_1 C_2 \hat{A}$

For example, Burt and Howard (1956) found the following correlations for IQ:

$$\text{between spouses } r_{SP} = 0.3875$$

$$\text{between parent/offspring } r_{P/O} = 0.4887$$

$$\text{between sibs } r_{S/S} = 0.5069$$

therefore:

$$C_1 C_2 = \frac{2(0.4887)}{1 + 0.3875}$$

$$= 0.7044$$

$$\hat{A} = 0.3875(0.7044)$$

$$= 0.2730$$

$$C_1 = 4(0.5069) - 0.7044(1 + 0.5460)$$

$$= 0.9386$$

Therefore the partition of the total variance is then:

1. *Environmental* $= 1 - 0.9386 = 0.0614$

2. *Non-environmental*
   (a) Non-additive (due to dominance)
   $$= 0.9386 - 0.7044 = 0.2342$$
   (b) Additive:
   expected under random mating
   $$= 0.7044(1 - 0.2730) = 0.5121$$
   due to assortative mating
   $$= 0.7044(0.2730) = 0.1923$$

Thus assortative mating can have a significant effect on the genetic variance. However, as Cavalli-Sforza and Bodmer (1971) point out, the real situation may well be more complicated than such simple models would lead us to believe.

The partition of variance has also been calculated for stature and total dermal ridge count (Table 3.1). In the latter trait, as one would expect, the contribution by assortative mating is very small and not significantly different from zero.

Table 3.1   Partition of variance determined from correlations between relatives for IQ, stature and total dermal ridge count

				Partition of variance (%)			
				Non-genetic	Genetic		
	Correlations				Non-additive	Additive	
	Spouses (r_{SP})	Parent-offspring $(r_{P/O})$	Sibs $(r_{S/S})$			Random mating	Assortative mating
IQ	0·39	0·49	0·51	7	23	51	19
Stature	0·28	0·51	0·54	—	21	62	17
Ridge count	0·05	0·48	0·50	—	9	87	4

Spuhler (1968) reported correlations between spouses for 105 physical characteristics. Apart from age, weight and stature, the majority of the correlations were less than 0·2 and many were less than 0·1.

Inbreeding

Two individuals are said to be *consanguineous* if they have at least one ancestor in common and, in practice, this common ancestor is usually considered to be no more remote than a great-great grand-parent. The offspring of consanguineous parents are by definition *inbred*.

Determination of the coefficient of inbreeding

The coefficient of inbreeding (F) may be defined as the probability that an individual (say C) will have, at a given locus, two genes identical by descent from a common ancestor. There are a number of ways in which it may be determined, the simplest being by path analysis or isonymy.

Path analysis. If n and n' are the number of generations in the lines of descent from a common ancester to the *parents* of individual C then

$$F = \Sigma \left(\frac{1}{2}\right)^{n+n'+1}$$

where summation is for each common ancestor.

Thus in the offspring of first cousins once removed (Fig. 3.2) the number of generations in line of descent from A to the mother is 3 (n), and to the father is 2 (n'). Similarly the number of generations in line of descent from B to the mother is 3 (n) and to the father is 2 (n'). Therefore:

$$F = \left(\frac{1}{2}\right)^6 + \left(\frac{1}{2}\right)^6$$

$$= \frac{1}{32}$$

In the case of X-linkage (Wright, 1922, 1950/1)

$$F = \sum \left(\frac{1}{2}\right)^{n_f}$$

where n_f = number of females in a line of descent and the summation relates to paths which have no male to male succession. A method for calculating the inbreeding coefficient for X-linked genes has been described in detail by Kudo and Sakaguchi (1963).

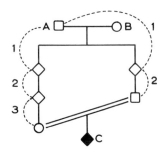

Fig. 3.2 Paths used in calculating 'F' of a child of parents who are first cousins once removed.

Isonymy. The coefficient of inbreeding can also be determined from the frequency of marriages between individuals with identical surnames (Crow and Mange, 1965) the reason being that in many societies the surname is transmitted in a regular pattern which closely corresponds to the biological ancestry. Now the frequency of isonymous pairs divided by four gives the inbreeding coefficient from random mating (F_r). Thus if:

p_i = proportion of males with a certain surname

q_i = proportion of females with a certain surname

then $F_r = \dfrac{\sum p_i q_i}{4}$

and $F = F_n + (1 - F_n)F_r$

and $F_n = \dfrac{P - \sum p_i q_i}{4(1 - \sum p_i q_i)}$

where P = observed proportion of isonymous marriages
F_r = inbreeding coefficient from *random* mating
F_n = inbreeding coefficient from *non-random* mating
F = total inbreeding coefficient.

Thus in a study of the Hutterites, a religious isolate in North America, there were 446 marriages between 1940–61 of which 87 were between individuals with the same surname. For example there were 30 males and 33 females with the surname 'Wi' therefore the *expected* number of marriages between these individuals with random mating is:

$$\left(\frac{30}{446}\right)\left(\frac{33}{446}\right)446$$

$$= 2{\cdot}22$$

whereas 5 such marriages were observed. In this way the total number of expected isonymous marriages with random mating was 79·55 whereas the observed number was 87.

Therefore the expected proportion of isonymous marriages was:

$$\frac{79{\cdot}55}{446}$$

$$= 0{\cdot}178$$

and therefore

$$F_r = \frac{0{\cdot}178}{4}$$

$$= 0{\cdot}0445$$

Now

$$P = \frac{87}{446}$$

$$= 0{\cdot}195$$

$$F_n = \frac{P - \sum p_i q_i}{4(1 - \sum p_i q_i)}$$

$$= \frac{0{\cdot}195 - 0{\cdot}178}{4(0{\cdot}822)}$$

$$= 0{\cdot}0052$$

Now

$$F = F_n + (1 - F_n)F_r$$
$$= 0.0052 + (1 - 0.0052)0.0445$$
$$= 0.0495$$

Thus the average relationship is equivalent to something between first cousins ($F = 1/16$ or 0.0625) and first cousins once removed ($F = 1/32$ or 0.0313). Almost the entire inbreeding effect is due to random marriages. The component from non-random marriages ($F_n = 0.0052$) is very small and not significantly different from zero.

The attraction of the isonymy method in estimating the coefficient of inbreeding is its simplicity. But the method should not be applied uncritically. For example, there may have been some duplication of surnames at the time the names were first introduced into the population, and assigning a family's name to an adopted child and giving any name other than the father's to an illegitimate child will affect the estimate of the coefficient of inbreeding from isonymy. Overall it seems likely that isonymy will tend to *overestimate* the actual amount of inbreeding in a given population.

It is of interest that surname has also been used as a 'genetic marker' in some studies (Ashley and Davies, 1966) though its value in this regard has yet to be fully assessed.

The amount of consanguinity in a population is best expressed as the *average inbreeding coefficient*

$$= \sum p_i F_i$$

where p_i is the proportion of marriages with inbreeding coefficient F_i. Thus in a study of consanguinity among French Canadians in the Province of Quebec (Laberge, 1966) out of a total of 96 marriages in the Isle aux Coudres in the Gulf of St. Lawrence, 13 were consanguineous (Table 3.2). In this study the overall average inbreeding coefficient in the Province was 0.0014.

Table 3.2   Average inbreeding coefficient in the Isle aux Coudres (Laberge, 1966)

	Total	1st cousin	1st cousin once removed	2nd cousin
No. of marriages	96	1	4	8
Proportion (p_i)	—	0.0104	0.0417	0.0833
Inbreeding (F_i)	—	0.0625	0.0313	0.0156
$p_i F_i$	—	0.00065	0.00131	0.00130
	$\sum p_i F_i = 0.0033$			

In most Western societies the average inbreeding coefficient is always less than 0.001 but in some isolated societies it may be greater than

0·04, but this is obviously influenced by marriage customs. Thus the coefficient of inbreeding is high in communities in Southern India because of preferential uncle–niece marriages, but is low in Eskimo communities because of taboos against inbreeding in any form.

The value, in practical terms, of estimating the coefficient of inbreeding is that it allows us to predict:

1. The incidence of a particular recessive disorder in an inbred population since this is equal to

$$Fq + q^2(1 - F)$$

Thus if the incidence of a recessive disorder in a randomly mating population is 1 in 10 000 ($q^2 = 0·0001$) then among marriages in an inbred population in which F is 0·04, the expected incidence (all else being equal) will be

$$(0·04)(0·01) + (0·0001)(0·96)$$

$$= 0·000496$$

or approximately 1 in 2000.

2. The proportion of heterozygotes for a particular recessive disorder in an inbred population since

$$H_F = (1 - F)H_o$$

where H_F and H_o denote the proportion of heterozygotes in populations with and without inbreeding.

3. The 'genetic load' (defined as the proportion of the population lost by selection), because certain components of the genetic load increase linearly with the coefficient of inbreeding. However in order to calculate the genetic load in this way it is necessary to know not only the value of F but also the fitness (see p. 28) of the various genotypes and apart from one or two disorders this is rarely known with any precision. The subject of genetic load has been interestingly discussed by Fraser and Mayo (1974).

The *coefficient of relationship* (R) is a measure of the degree of genetic relationship between two individuals and may be defined as the probability that both possess an identical gene by descent from a common ancestor(s). It is equal to (1/2) to the power of the number of generations in the lines of descent from a common ancestor(s) to the individuals whose coefficient of relationship is being determined:

$$R = \Sigma \left(\frac{1}{2}\right)^{n+n'}$$

or
$$R = 2F$$

That is the inbreeding coefficient of a child is half the coefficient of

relationship of its parents. Some values of F and R ar
Table 3.3.

Table 3.3 Coefficients of inbreeding (F) and relationship (R) ar
probability of isonymy (P) for various consanguineous matings

Mating	F	R	P
Sibs	1/4	1/2	1
Uncle–neice, aunt–nephew	1/8	1/4	1/2
1st cousins	1/16	1/8	1/4
1st cousins once removed	1/32	1/16	1/8
2nd cousins	1/64	1/32	1/16
2nd cousins once removed	1/128	1/64	1/32
3rd cousins	1/256	1/128	1/64

Cousin marriages

With rare recessive traits, the parents of affected individuals are often
related, the reason being that such individuals are more likely to carry
the same genes because they have inherited them from a common
ancestor. In fact the chance that first cousins will carry the same gene
is 1 in 8. The frequency (C) of first-cousin marriages among the
parents of children with any particular autosomal recessive disorder is
(Dahlberg, 1947)

$$C = \frac{a(1 + 15q)}{a + 16q - aq}$$

where a = frequency of 1st cousin marriages in the general population.

If 'q' is very small then approximately

$$C = \frac{a}{a + 16q}$$

Alternatively if the frequency of first-cousin marriages in the general
population (a) and among parents of affected children (C) are known
then the gene frequency can be estimated since

$$q = \frac{a(1 - C)}{16C - Ca - 15a}$$

Some examples of recessive disorders and the approximate frequencies
of consanguinity among the parents are given in Table 3.4, where it is
assumed that the frequency of first-cousin marriages in the general
population is about 1 in 200. Note that the rarer a recessive disorder
the more likely are the parents to be related. An increase in consanguinity among the parents of children with a particular rare disorder
may therefore be used as evidence that the disorder is inherited as a
recessive trait.

Table 3.4 Prevalence of first-cousin marriages among the parents of individuals with various recessive disorders

Disorder	Frequency of homozygotes (q^2)	Gene frequency (q)	% Consanguinity* (1)	(2)
Alkaptonuria	1/1 000 000	0·0010	24·2	23·8
Cystinuria	1/100 000	0·0032	9·3	8·9
Albinism	1/20 000	0·0071	4·7	4·2
Phenylketonuria	1/15 000	0·0082	4·1	3·7
Fibrocystic disease	1/2000	0·0224	1·8	1·4

* Consanguinity estimated from (1) $\dfrac{a(1 + 15q)}{a + 16q - aq}$ (2) $\dfrac{a}{a + 16q}$

Gene flow

Another process by which genetic variation is introduced into a population is by gene flow. That is when individuals from outside the population contribute to the gene pool either by *migration* or *racial admixture*. Migration may result in a gene being spread in one direction only and the frequency gradient that may result is referred to as a *cline*. Thus the frequency of the gene for blood group B is very high in Asia (over 25 per cent) but gradually decreases as one travels westward across Europe until in Britain, France and Scandinavia it is less than 10 per cent. It has been suggested that this gradient or cline is the consequence of invasions by Mongoloids who pushed westward from about A.D. 500 until A.D. 1500. Miscegenation between the invaders and the native population in which blood group B was rare or absent, led to the diffusion of the B gene across Europe (Candela, 1942). Of course it is equally possible that this gradient in the frequency of blood group B gene might have been the result of some as yet unknown selective force which followed a similar geographic gradient.

Gene flow may also mean *admixture* of two or more genetically dissimilar populations so creating a hybrid group, for example, the racial admixture which resulted in the United States from miscegenation between African Negroes and American Whites or in Hawaii between Polynesians, Asiatics and Europeans.

If '*m*' is the proportion of genes at a particular locus in a hybrid population (*H*) which is derived from a population (*P*) which has miscegenated with an immigrant population (*I*), and if q is the gene frequency, then

$$q_H = mq_P + (1 - m)q_I$$

and therefore

$$m = \frac{|q_H - q_I|^*}{|q_P - q_I|}$$

* The vertical lines mean the *absolute* values of the differences, that is the differences are always positive.

This is sometimes referred to as *Bernstein's* equation. If the gene in question is absent from the immigrant population then

$$m = \frac{q_H}{q_P}$$

In studying the problem of gene flow in relation to the American Negro, Reed (1969) considered the Duffy blood group ($Fy(a+)$) a good marker in this regard. Thus the mean frequency of Fy^a gene in West Africa (I) is at most 0·030, in American whites (P) is 0·429, and in American Negroes (H), in southern California, is about 0·094, therefore

$$m = \frac{q_H - q_I}{q_P - q_I}$$
$$= \frac{0·094 - 0·030}{0·429 - 0·030}$$
$$= 0·160$$

If however one assumes that Fy^a might well have been absent from the original African population, then

$$m = \frac{q_H}{q_P}$$
$$= \frac{0·094}{0·429}$$
$$= 0·219$$

Thus from the evidence of Fy^a gene of the Duffy blood group system, the proportion of American Negro genes which are of American white origin is between 16 and 22 per cent in southern California. In contrast the proportion is less than 4 per cent in Charleston, South Carolina which probably reflects cultural barriers to gene flow.

It should be noted however, that in estimating 'm' in this way, several assumptions are made (Workman, Blumberg and Cooper, 1963). It is assumed that the deviation of q_H from q_I is solely due to gene flow. It disregards the possible effects of natural selection which can introduce a serious bias. Reed (1969) chose the Duffy blood group system because there was no obvious evidence of strong selection at this locus in Californian Negroes, at least as shown from studies of fetal and infant growth and viability and from adult growth and fertility. It also assumes that there is no assortative or preferential mating between the two populations. Such calculations also depend on the estimation of gene frequencies in the original populations and in the present hybrid population.

Finally it should be noted that gene flow is also related to the effective size of a population (N_e) and the coefficient of inbreeding (F). That is

$$F = \frac{1}{4N_em + 1}$$

therefore

$$m = \frac{1 - F}{4N_eF}$$

Thus in the Dunkers, a religious isolate in the United States, F was estimated to be 0·0254 and N_e to be 90 (see p. 12), and therefore

$$m = \frac{1 - 0·0254}{4(90)(0·0254)}$$

$$= 0·1066$$

which represents the gene flow into the isolate each generation (Glass et al., 1952).

Selection

Selection has been studied more than perhaps any other aspect of human population genetics. The subject is discussed in detail elsewhere (for example Fisher, 1930; Spuhler, 1963; Bajema, 1971; Roberts, 1975), and here we shall only be concerned with how selection forces, in relation to human disease, can be measured.

Selection forces may be either natural or artificial. The former occurs under natural conditions without the intervention of man, whereas the latter is a direct consequence of man's intervention by introducing effective treatments for otherwise lethal disorders or limiting the reproduction of persons with hereditary defects. Selection forces operate at all stages of development though in humans this is usually considered in relation to postnatal development and may operate through differential mortality or differential fertility.

Selection forces disturb the Hardy-Weinberg equilibrium by increasing or decreasing fitness. In this sense fitness has a very special meaning and will be discussed later (p. 28).

The *coefficient of selection* (s) may be defined as the proportional reduction in the gametic contribution of a particular genotype to the next generation. If f is fitness

$$s = 1 - f$$

It can be shown that at equilibrium for an autosomal recessive trait

$$s = \frac{\mu}{q^2}$$

for a rare autosomal dominant trait

$$s = \frac{\mu}{q}$$

and for an X-linked recessive trait, in males

$$s = \frac{3\mu}{q}$$

where μ = mutation rate.

Heterozygote advantage in recessive disorders
The estimation of 's' has mainly been of interest in autosomal recessive disorders in which the apparent high frequency of affected individuals cannot be accounted for by mutation alone or genetic heterogeneity (due to different loci or multiple alleles at the same locus) and therefore it is postulated that the heterozygote may have some selective advantage. Thus the Hardy-Weinberg equilibrium is modified to

$$f_1 p^2 + f_2 2pq + f_3 q^2$$

where f_1, f_2 and f_3 are the relative fitnesses of the three genotypes.
When a stable equilibrium is maintained by selection such that the heterozygote is 'superior' to either homozygote ($f_2 > f_1$ and f_3) this is sometimes referred to as *over-dominance*.
If the coefficients of selection in the normal homozygote and affected homozygote are s_1 and s_2 respectively then in either the entire population, in the case of an autosomal recessive disorder, or among females in the case of an X-linked recessive disorder:

	Genotypes			
	AA	Aa	aa	Total
Initial population	p^2	$2pq$	q^2	1
After selection	$p^2(1-s_1)$	$2pq$	$q^2(1-s_2)$	$1 - p^2 s_1 - q^2 s_2 = T$
Relative contribution to next generation	$\dfrac{p^2(1-s_1)}{T}$	$\dfrac{2pq}{T}$	$\dfrac{q^2(1-s_2)}{T}$	1

Therefore in the next generation

$$q_{n+1} = \tfrac{1}{2}(Aa) + (aa)$$

$$= \frac{pq + q^2(1-s_2)}{T}$$

$$= \frac{q - q^2 s_2}{T}$$

Therefore the change in gene frequency

$$= q_{n+1} - q$$

$$= \frac{q - q^2 s_2}{T} - q$$

$$= \frac{pq(ps_1 - qs_2)}{T}$$

But at equilibrium the change in gene frequency from one generation to another is zero. That is when

$$ps_1 = qs_2$$

$$(1 - q)s_1 = qs_2$$

$$s_1 - qs_1 = qs_2$$

$$q = \frac{s_1}{s_1 + s_2}$$

If, as in many serious recessive disorders, the rare homozygote is so severely affected as not to survive to have children or survives but is infertile then $s_2 = 1$ and

$$q = \frac{1}{s_1 + 1}$$

and therefore

$$s_1 = \frac{q}{1 - q}$$

Thus in the case of fibrocystic disease ($q^2 = 1/2000$: $q = 0.022$) $s_1 = 0.022/0.978$ or 0.0225. To maintain the present frequency of this disease the heterozygote must therefore have a fitness of 2·25 per cent greater than the normal homozygote. To demonstrate a relative increase in fitness of this order of magnitude in heterozygotes would be very difficult but attempts have been made. For example in fibrocystic disease (Danks, Allan and Anderson, 1965; Knudson, Wayne and Hallett, 1967), Tay-Sachs disease (Myrianthopoulos and Aronson, 1966) and phenylketonuria (Woolf *et al.*, 1975). How this is done will be discussed later (p. 28). The relationship between the frequency of affecteds ($q^2\%$) and heterozygote advantage is given in Figure 3.3.

Heterozygous advantage may well have played a part in determining the relatively high incidences in certain populations of sickle-cell anaemia and perhaps β-thalassaemia, in these cases through an increased resistance to falciparum malaria (Allison, 1964). The high incidence of some other disorders (Table 3.5) might also be due to

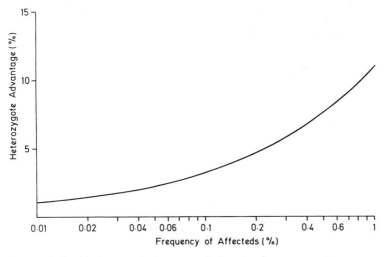

Fig. 3.3 Relationship between the frequency of affecteds (q^2 per cent) and heterozygote advantage (per cent).

heterozygous advantage but may be partly related to population size in former times in which mutation could have played a greater role in determining gene frequencies (Mayo, 1970). It is also possible that the so-called *founder effect* may have been important in certain circumstances as in the case of the high incidence of Tay-Sachs disease in a non-Jewish semi-isolate in North America (Kelly *et al.*, 1975). Alternative explanations for some of these high gene frequencies are close linkage to genes whose alleles have been favoured by selection (*hitchhiker* effect) or epistatic interaction with an unlinked gene (Wagener and Cavalli-Sforza, 1975).

Table 3.5   Estimated heterozygous advantage (in the absence of other factors) in maintaining the frequencies of certain recessive disorders in which it is presumed in earlier times, without treatment, most homozygous affecteds would not have survived to have children

Disorder	Location	Frequency of affecteds (q^2)	Gene frequency (q)	Heterozygous advantage (%)
Sickle-cell anaemia	Africa	1/25	0·200	25·0
β-Thalassaemia	Mediterranean	1/200	0·071	7·6
Fibrocystic disease	Europe	1/2000	0·022	2·2
Tay-Sachs disease	Ashkenazi Jews	1/3600	0·017	1·7
Phenylketonuria	Europe	1/15 000	0·008	0·8
	Ireland and West Scotland	1/5000	0·014	1·4

Equations relating gene frequencies to coefficients of selection under various conditions are summarized in Table 3.6.

Table 3.6 Summary of equations relating gene frequencies to coefficients of selection under various circumstances

Selection against	Initial fitnesses			Equilibrium
	AA (p^2)	Aa $(2pq)$	aa (q^2)	
AA and aa	$1 - s_1$	1	$1 - s_2$	$q = \dfrac{s_1}{s_1 + s_2}$
AA and Aa	$1 - s$ (rare)	$1 - s$	1	$q \simeq \dfrac{\mu}{s}$
aa	1	1	$1 - s$ (rare)	$q = \sqrt{\dfrac{\mu}{s}}$

Estimation of fitness

We have seen that it is possible to estimate the coefficient of selection from gene frequencies. It can also be estimated directly by determining the fitness of various genotypes.

Biological or Darwinian fitness is a measure of the extent to which an individual with a mutant gene can reproduce so that the gene is maintained in the population. It is not synonymous with fertility *per se* since any offspring who die before reaching maturity will not contribute at all to the next generation. The subject, and some of the problems involved in estimating fitness have been discussed in non-mathematical terms by Clarke (1959b). Biological fitness has been variously expressed as:

1. The total number of offspring (excluding stillbirths and abortions)
2. The number of offspring who reach reproductive age (say 20).
3. The number of offspring who reach the mean age at which the parents reproduced
4. The number of offspring who complete their reproductive life (say 45).

Method three is the ideal but it is often not easy to determine because in most family studies there is insufficient data. For this reason investigators often rely on the first method.

Comparisons are usually made with comparable data (similar age and sex) from the general population or normal sibs. However, fertility is affected by many factors other than genetic including race, period of time and social class, etc. It is therefore not easy in practice to obtain a value for a general population which is strictly comparable with affected individuals. Statistical procedures have been developed for getting round these problems but they are complex and require extensive demographic data (Reed, 1959; Charlesworth and Charlesworth, 1973).

For this reason some investigators have made comparisons with normal sibs. However, sibs of affected individuals are not always representative of the general population. Further, apparently normal sibs may in fact be carriers of the gene and subsequently develop the disease if onset is not necessarily in early life. They may also have not completed their reproductive life at the time of the study.

When there is variable age at death in affected individuals whose fitness is to be assessed, a simple approach is to determine the number of offspring per number of reproductive years (say 20 to 45). Thus in a study of benign Becker type X-linked muscular dystrophy the mean number of live births per 100 fertile years was 4·959 for affected males and 7·418 for their unaffected male sibs. The relative fitness is therefore 0·67. It should be noted that in this disease one can be certain that sibs are in fact normal by determining their serum level of creatine kinase.

Another common problem has been to assess the relative fitness of heterozygotes for severe recessive disorders in order to determine if there is any heterozygous advantage (see p. 26). In this situation there is the problem that if one considers the offspring of two heterozygous parents, such matings will have been ascertained in the first place because they have produced an affected child and this might well have biased their plans for further children. Also they will have had to have had at least one child.

There are essentially two ways of dealing with these problems. Firstly, one may consider the reproductive performance of the *grand-parents* of affected children since at least one maternal and one paternal grandparent will be unsuspecting heterozygotes, but comparisons must be made with comparable controls of the same generation. Such an approach has been made, for example, in the case of fibrocystic disease (Danks *et al.*, 1965; Knudson *et al.*, 1967) and Tay-Sachs disease (Myrianthopoulos and Aronson, 1966).

Alternatively one can study the reproductive performance of couples who are both heterozygotes by determining the number and outcome of pregnancies *previous* to the affected child, as was done by Woolf *et al.* (1975) in the case of phenylketonuria, or by making special allowances for the various biases which may be present (Oakes, 1968). Here one takes as controls, families with at least one child and the mean family size of such families is then calculated. The mean family size of families with two heterozygous parents and at least one affected child is then determined from which it is possible to derive a value for '*s*'. (Tables for doing these various calculations are given by Oakes, 1968.) This method however, assumes that there has been *complete* ascertainment of all cases in a particular population and this might be quite impractical.

Tanaka (1974) has devised a very simple and effective way of estimating fitness. He has shown that

$$f = \frac{A_p}{A_o}$$

where A_p = frequency of the trait among *parents* of index cases
and A_o = frequency of the trait among *offspring* of index cases

The underlying principle is that, if selection against a specific disorder is sufficiently strong then the frequency of affected individuals among parents of index cases will be lower than among the offspring of index cases, and this reduction is proportional to the intensity of selection. The method is widely applicable but is particularly valuable in autosomal dominant and multifactorial disorders. Tanaka gives worked examples for a number of disorders. For example, in one study of schizophrenia A_p = 4·38 per cent, A_o = 12·31 per cent and therefore $f = 0·36$; and in one study of neurofibromatosis A_p = 18·27 per cent, A_o = 35·23 per cent and therefore $f = 0·52$.

Unfortunately the method is not particularly suitable for rare autosomal recessive or X-linked recessive disorders because A_o is too small to be estimated precisely. Further, the method is only valid if the frequency of the disorder is roughly the same in both the parent and offspring generations. In some disorders, because of changes in accepted diagnostic criteria over the last few decades, this may present an important objection to the method.

Finally, before leaving the subject, it should be noted that fitness may not always be reduced. In Huntington's chorea, for example, evidence suggests that affected individuals are in fact more fecund than their normal sibs and members of the general population of comparable age. In one study fitness in Huntington's chorea was estimated to be 1·14 compared with the general population (Shokeir, 1975). If maintained this would result in a steady increase in the incidence of the disorder in future generations.

Fitness and incidence of X-linked disorders

In X-linked recessive disorders knowing the fitness of affected males (f), and if the fitness of carrier females is 1·0, then it is possible to determine the incidence of affected males (I) and carrier females (H) in terms of the mutation rate* since at equilibrium

$$I = \mu + H/2$$

and $$H = 2\mu + H/2 + If$$

In a condition such as Duchenne muscular dystrophy (and many other serious X-linked recessive disorders) where $f = 0$ then

$$H = 2\mu + H/2$$

and therefore $$H = 4\mu$$

and since $$I = \mu + H/2$$

$$I = 3\mu$$

* Assuming the mutation rate is the same in males and females.

In Becker type muscular dystrophy an approximate value of f is 0·70. Therefore

$$H = 2\mu + H/2 + I(0·7)$$

but $\qquad\qquad I = \mu + H/2$

substituting for I,

then $\qquad\qquad H = 2\mu + H/2 + (\mu + H/2)0·7$

therefore $\qquad\qquad H = 18\mu$

and $\qquad\qquad I = 10\mu$

Values for H and I for some other disorders are given in Table 3.7. These results have important implications in probability calculations for genetic counselling (see p. 93).

Table 3.7   The incidence of affected males and carrier females in terms of the mutation rate (μ) in X-linked recessive disorders where the fitness in carrier females is assumed to be 1·0.

Fitness of affected males	Incidence (times μ)		Example
	Affected males	Carrier females	
0·0	3	4	⎰Duchenne muscular dystrophy ⎱Lesch-Nyhan syndrome, etc.
0·1	3·4	4·7	—
0·2	3·8	5·5	—
0·3*	4·3	6·6	Neonatal hypoparathyroidism
0·4*	5	8	Vitamin D resistant rickets
0·5	6	10	—
0·6*	7·5	13	Anhidrotic ectodermal dysplasia
0·7	10	18	⎰Becker muscular dystrophy ⎱Haemophilia A
0·8*	15	28	Diabetes insipidus, pituitary type
0·9	30	58	—

* From data in Stevenson and Kerr (1967).

Mutation

The Hardy-Weinberg equilibrium depends on a constant rate of mutation, but clearly this may be increased by exposure to X-radiation or mutagenic chemicals. In discussing mutation this usually infers gene or so-called 'point' mutation though it should be remembered that chromosomal rearrangements are also a form of mutation. There are two methods for determining mutation rates: direct and indirect.

Direct method for estimating mutation rates

This method is only applicable to autosomal dominant traits which are rare and always fully penetrant and X-linked recessive disorders when the carrier state is detectable. An example of the former is provided by a study of achondroplasia.

Summarizing the results of several recent newborn surveys, Gardner (1976) found 6 cases of *true* achondroplasia of normal parents out of a total of 227 339 live births. However in each affected child the mutation could have occurred in either the gene supplied by the mother or that supplied by the father. Therefore the mutation rate *per gene*

$$= 6/2(227\,339)$$
$$= 13 \cdot 2 \times 10^{-6}$$

the standard error of which is

$$= \sqrt{\frac{pq}{2N}}$$
$$= \sqrt{\frac{0 \cdot 0000132 \times 0 \cdot 9999868}{454\,678}}$$
$$= 5 \cdot 4 \times 10^{-6}$$

Therefore the mutation rate for achondroplasia may be expressed as $13 \cdot 2 \pm 5 \cdot 4 \times 10^{-6}$.

The application of the direct method to an X-linked recessive disorder where it is possible to detect the carrier state, is illustrated in the case of Duchenne muscular dystrophy (DMD) in which a proportion of healthy female carriers have a raised serum level of creatine kinase. In one study (Gardner-Medwin, 1970), 22 out of 35 known carriers had raised serum levels of creatine kinase. Of 56 mothers of sporadic cases, 15 had raised levels. Thus the proportion of new mutations (mothers are non-carriers) among sporadic cases is $[56 - (35/22)15]/56$ or $0 \cdot 574$. Now over a 9 year period (1952–1960) 43 *sporadic* cases were born and therefore the number of new mutations is $(43)(0 \cdot 574)$ or $24 \cdot 682$. The total number of males born in this period who survived to age 5 (by which time almost all cases of DMD are diagnosed) was 236 200. Thus the mutation rate is $24 \cdot 682/236\,200$ or $10 \cdot 5 \times 10^{-5}$. Thus if '$P$' is the proportion of sporadic cases presumed to be due to new mutations and if in a given period 'n' is the number of sporadic cases and 'N' the total male births, the mutation rate is equal to

$$Pn/N$$

The direct method of estimating mutation rates is not applicable to recessive traits since a mutation to a recessive gene will go unrecognized if the mutant gene is completely recessive and not manifest in the heterozygote. The method is most useful in relatively severe dominant disorders in which affected individuals often do not have offspring, so that a significant proportion of affected persons are likely to be the result of new mutations. In other situations the so-called *indirect* method is used.

Indirect method for estimating mutation rates

In dominant disorders if μ is the mutation rate (per gene per generation) then the frequency of cases due to fresh mutations is 2μ. If the reproductive fitness is 'f' and the incidence (p. 121) of the disorder is 'I' then in each generation the number of cases eliminated is

$$= (1 - f)I$$

In a state of equilibrium where the frequency of the condition does not change from generation to generation, then the number of cases arising as a result of new mutations must be equal to the number being eliminated because of reduced fitness. Thus

$$2\mu = I(1 - f)$$

and therefore

$$\mu = \tfrac{1}{2}I(1 - f)$$

Similarly it can be shown that for an autosomal recessive trait

$$\mu = I(1 - f)$$

for an X-linked dominant trait

$$\mu = \tfrac{2}{3}I(1 - f)$$

for an X-linked recessive trait

$$\mu = \tfrac{1}{3}I'(1 - f)$$

and for an holandric trait

$$\mu = I'(1 - f)$$

In the latter two cases I' represents the incidence of affected males among all males whereas I represents the incidence of affected males and females in the total population. The term $(1 - f)$ is referred to as the coefficient of selection (s) against the gene (p. 24).

It should be remembered that there are a number of problems and sources of error in estimating mutation rates by both the direct or indirect methods. Spuriously high estimates will be obtained if clinically similar but genetically different disorders are lumped together. Another problem is that both methods depend upon the accurate determination of the incidence of the disorder in the general population and this may be difficult to obtain. Further, the incidence of a disorder in a particular population may be affected by factors other than selection and mutation, i.e. by inbreeding, genetic drift, founder effect, etc. Finally, the indirect method depends on the estimation of fitness of affected individuals and this poses special problems (p. 28). The subject of spontaneous mutation in man has been critically and interestingly reviewed by Vogel and Rathenberg (1975) where the reader will find the subject dealt with in detail.

4. Segregation Analysis

To test a particular genetic hypothesis in experimental animals one studies the progeny of controlled matings. This, of course, is not possible in human populations and the geneticist has to approach the problem indirectly by fitting probability models to family data: that is by comparing the observed proportion of affected sibs and offspring with the proportion expected according to a particular genetic hypothesis. This is referred to as *segregation analysis*. The main problems of such studies arise through the different methods of *ascertaining* families and affected individuals, and through pooling data from different families which is necessary because no single family is ever large enough to test a given genetic hypothesis. Various statistical methods have been developed in order to eliminate such biases, but it should be remembered that segregation analysis may also be complicated by factors inherent in the data itself such as incomplete families, inaccurate diagnoses and genetic heterogeneity. It therefore behoves the Medical Geneticist to consider these possibilities carefully before attempting to combine data from different families and applying the methods of segregation analysis.

Autosomal dominant inheritance

To determine if a particular characteristic is inherited as an autosomal dominant trait, the number of affected offspring of an affected parent with a healthy spouse is compared with the expected number using χ^2 test. Thus in one study of opalescent dentine, out of a total of 112 offspring of affected parents, 52 were similarly affected whereas 56 would have been expected assuming simple dominant inheritance (Neel and Schull, 1954):

Offspring	Normal	Affected	Total
observed	60	52	112
expected	56	56	112
$(O - E)^2$	16	16	—
$\dfrac{(O - E)^2}{E}$	0·286	0·286	0·572

Thus χ^2 is 0·572. With one degree of freedom (p. 6) to be significant χ^2 should exceed 3·841 (see Appendix 2, p. 132). The value obtained is less than this and therefore there is no significant departure from the expected number of normal and affected offspring assuming autosomal dominant inheritance.

The significance of a departure from an expected ratio of 1 : 1 among the offspring of affected parents can be calculated quite simply from the formula given by Roberts (1973):

$$\chi^2 = \frac{[(A - N) - 1]^2}{A + N}$$

where
A = total number of affected offspring
N = total number of normal offspring

The subtraction of unity from the difference in the numerator is Yates' correction which has to be included when dealing with small numbers. Thus if there were 15 affected and 12 normal offspring in a number of families in each of which one of the parents was affected then

$$\chi^2 = \frac{[(15 - 12) - 1]^2}{27}$$

$$= \frac{4}{27}$$

$$= 0 \cdot 148$$

In this example, therefore, there is no significant departure from the expected 1 : 1 ratio among the offspring in the families studied.

It should be remembered that in testing for autosomal dominant inheritance, families should be ascertained irrespective of the nature of the offspring of affected individuals, i.e. never because there are affected children in the families.

Autosomal recessive inheritance

The situation is more complicated when testing for autosomal recessive inheritance. Matings between heterozygous parents are ascertained only because they have produced affected children, however, by chance, some families where both parents are heterozygous will produce only normal children (heterozygotes and normal homozygotes) and will therefore not be detected. By selecting only families which produce affected children a bias is introduced which will result in a spuriously high proportion of affected individuals in such families. Secondly, the more affected children there are in a given sibship the more likely it is that the sibship will be ascertained. Thus the manner in which families are ascertained is critically important in testing for recessive inheritance and determines the method of analysis to be used.

There are three ways in which families may be ascertained:

1. An exhaustive search may be made to ascertain every affected individual in the community regardless of whether or not there are any affected relatives (= *complete ascertainment*). In practice, it is often impossible to ascertain every case in the community in which case ascertainment is referred to as being *incomplete*.

2. Each family may have been ascertained through one, and only one, affected individual irrespective of how many affected children there may be in the family (= *single incomplete ascertainment*).

3. Some families may have been ascertained more than once through different affected sibs, i.e. there may be more than one proband per sibship (= *multiple incomplete ascertainment*).

The methods of analysis, depending on the mode of ascertainment, may be summarized as follows:

> 1. *Complete* (= *truncate*) *ascertainment*
>   (a) *A priori* (= direct or Apert) method
>   (b) Maximum likelihood method
>   (c) 'Singles' method
> 2. *Single incomplete ascertainment*
>   'Sib' method
> 3. *Multiple incomplete ascertainment*
>   'Proband' method

Thus the investigator should be quite clear how families and affected individuals have been ascertained and then apply the method appropriate to the mode of ascertainment. Detailed discussions of some of these methods together with references to earlier work are given by Steinberg (1959).

Complete ascertainment

A priori method (*Hogben, 1931 ; 1946*). The actual number of affected individuals is compared with the number expected calculated from the truncate binomial

$$\sum \frac{sp}{1 - q^s} \cdot n_s$$

which has a variance of

$$\sum \left[\frac{spq}{1 - q^s} - \frac{s^2 p^2 q^s}{(1 - q^s)^2} \right] n_s$$

where
s = sibship size
n_s = number of sibships of size s
p = theoretical proportion, i.e. 0·25
$q = 1 - p$

Values for these two equations for various sibship sizes are given in Table 4.3 (p. 39).

For this method of analysis it is assumed that all cases in a given community have been ascertained. In practice, this is rarely possible but an exception would be the situation when every case of a rare disorder is studied in a well defined and relatively small community.

An example of this approach would be the reported study of the so-called Mast syndrome (a form of presenile dementia with motor disturbance) among the Amish, a religious isolate in the United States (Cross and McKusick, 1967).

The data from this study are summarized in Table 4.1.

Table 4.1 Sibships in which one or more persons with the Mast syndrome were offspring of unaffected parents. Individuals who died prior to age 12 have been excluded because of uncertainty as to their genotype.

Family	Affected	Normal	Total	No. of 'singles'
1	1	5	6	1
2	1	1	2	1
3	4	3	7	—
4	4	7	11	—
5	2	6	8	—
6	3	4	7	—
7	1	7	8	1
8	2	4	6	—
9	1	5	6	1
Totals	19	42	61	4

To apply the *a priori* method of analysis the data are set-out as shown in Table 4.2.

Table 4.2 The observed and expected numbers of affected individuals with the Mast syndrome assuming complete ascertainment.

Size of sibship s	No. of sibships n_s	Total no. of individuals $s \cdot n_s$	No. of affected individuals observed	No. of affected individuals expected	Variance
2	1	2	1	1·1428	0·1224
6	3	18	4	5·4744	2·3278
7	2	14	7	4·0392	1·9405
8	2	16	3	4·4450	2·3448
11	1	11	4	2·8710	1·8053
Totals	9	61	19	17·9724	8·5408
					s.e. = 2·9225

The expected numbers of affecteds and the variances are calculated in the following manner. In the case of sibships of size 6 ($s = 6$), there are 3 ($n_s = 3$) of these and therefore from the data in Table 4.3 the expected number of affected individuals in these sibships is

$$\frac{sp}{1-q^s} \cdot n_s$$

$$= (1 \cdot 8248)3$$

$$= 5 \cdot 4744$$

and the variance is

$$(0 \cdot 77595)3$$

$$= 2 \cdot 3278$$

Table 4.3 Values of $sp/1 - q^s$ and its variance for various sibship sizes (s) (*From* Hogben, L., 1946)

s	$p = 1/4$ and $q = 3/4$		$p = 1/2 = q$	
	$\dfrac{sp}{1-q^s}$	Variance	$\dfrac{sp}{1-q^s}$	Variance
1	1·000	0·0000	1·000	0·000
2	1·1428	0·12245	1·333	0·2222
3	1·2973	0·26297	1·715	0·4898
4	1·4628	0·42005	2·134	0·7822
5	1·6389	0·50178	2·581	1·082
6	1·8248	0·77595	3·047	1·379
7	2·0196	0·97024	3·527	1·667
8	2·2225	1·1724	4·015	1·945
9	2·4328	1·3802	4·509	2·215
10	2·649	1·5917	5·005	2·478
11	2·871	1·8053	5·503	2·737
12	3·098	2·0196	6·001	2·992
13	3·329	2·2335	6·5	3·245
14	3·563	2·4464	7·0	3·497
15	3·801	2·6575	7·5	3·748
16	4·041	2·8667	8·0	3·999
17	4·282	3·0738	8·5	4·249
18	4·525	3·2787	9·0	4·500
19	4·770	3·4814	9·5	4·75
20	5·016	3·6821	10·0	5·00

From the data in Table 4.2 it will be seen that the observed number of affected individuals differs from the expected number by 1·0276 which is 0·3516 times the standard error. Thus there is close agreement between the observed and expected numbers of affected sibs assuming autosomal recessive inheritance ($p = 0·25$). Tables (see p. 41) are also available which give values for $sp/1 - q^s$ for various values of $p = 0·15$ to $p = 0·35$ (Li, 1961).

Maximum likelihood method (Haldane, 1938). In this method no prior assumption is made regarding a value for 'p', i.e. 0·25 if testing for recessive inheritance. Instead the maximum likelihood estimate of 'p' is determined where

$$\frac{R}{p} = \sum \frac{sn_s}{1 - q^s}$$

which has a variance of

$$\sum \frac{pq(1 - q^s)^2}{sn_s(1 - q^s - spq^{s-1})}$$

where

    R = number of affected individuals in all sibships
    s = sibship size
    n_s = number of sibships of size 's'

the first equation being solved for 'p' by iteration.

To apply the maximum likelihood method of analysis the data are set out as in Table 4.4.

Table 4.4 The observed and expected numbers of affected individuals with the Mast syndrome when $p = 0·25$ and $p = 0·275$

Size of sibship s	No. of sibships n_s	No. of affected individuals			Reciprocal of variance†	
		observed	expected*			
			$p = 0·250$	$p = 0·275$	$p = 0·250$	$p = 0·275$
2	1	1	1·143	1·159	3·483	3·371
6	3	4	5·475	5·790	66·213	64·782
7	2	7	4·040	4·304	55·196	53·960
8	2	3	4·446	4·764	66·694	65·096
11	1	4	2·871	3·116	51·350	49·722
Totals	9	19	17·975	19·133	242·936	236·931

* $n_s \times$ values for $p = 0·250$ and $p = 0·275$ in Table 4.5A
† $n_s \times$ values for $p = 0·250$ and $p = 0·275$ in Table 4.5B.

A trial value of $p = 0·250$ is first chosen. This gives an expected number of affecteds of 17·975 (slightly different from Table 4.2 because of differences in the values of $sp/1 - q^s$ in Table 4.5A due to rounding-off). This is less than the observed number (i.e. 19). Therefore a greater value of 'p' is chosen. When $p = 0·275$, the expected number of affecteds is 19·133 which is slightly greater than the observed number. Thus 'p' must lie somewhere between 0·250 and 0·275. By linear interpolation when there are 19 affected individuals the corresponding value of 'p' is 0·272. Similarly by linear interpolation when $p = 0·272$ then the reciprocal of the variance is 237·6. The variance is therefore

$$1/237·6 = 0·00421$$

and the standard error is

$$\sqrt{0.00421} = 0.0649$$

The final result may be stated as

$$p = 0.272 \pm 0.065.$$

The reciprocal of the variance is given in Table 4.5B merely for convenience in order to avoid a lot of zeros if the variance itself were used. Thus when $s = 15$ and $p = 0.250$ then the variance is 0.01323.

Table 4.5A Values of $sp/1 - q^s$ for various values of 'p' and sibships of size 's' (*From* Li, C. C., 1961)

s	$p = 0.15$	$p = 0.20$	$p = 0.225$	$p = 0.25$	$p = 0.275$	$p = 0.30$	$p = 0.35$
2	1·081	1·111	1·127	1·143	1·159	1·176	1·212
3	1·666	1·230	1·263	1·297	1·333	1·370	1·448
4	1·255	1·355	1·408	1·463	1·520	1·579	1·704
5	1·348	1·487	1·562	1·639	1·719	1·803	1·980
6	1·445	1·626	1·723	1·825	1·930	2·040	2·271
7	1·545	1·772	1·893	2·020	2·152	2·288	2·576
8	1·649	1·923	2·069	2·223	2·382	2·547	2·892
9	1·757	2·079	2·252	2·433	2·620	2·814	3·217
10	1·868	2·241	2·441	2·649	2·865	3·087	3·548
11	1·982	2·407	2·635	2·871	3·116	3·367	3·884
12	2·098	2·577	2·833	3·098	3·371	3·651	4·224
13	2·218	2·751	3·035	3·329	3·631	3·938	4·567
14	2·341	2·929	3·241	3·563	3·893	4·229	4·912
15	2·465	3·109	3·450	3·801	4·158	4·521	5·258

Table 4.5B Reciprocal of variances for various values of 'p' and sibships of size 's' (*From* Li, C. C., 1961)

s	$p = 0.15$	$p = 0.20$	$p = 0.225$	$p = 0.25$	$p = 0.275$	$p = 0.30$	$p = 0.35$
2	4·583	3·858	3·640	3·483	3·371	3·295	3·229
3	9·600	8·188	7·774	7·480	7·278	7·149	7·061
4	15·038	12·967	12·367	11·948	11·665	11·489	11·386
5	20·882	18·163	17·380	16·833	16·463	16·230	16·077
6	27·113	23·739	22·761	22·071	21·594	21·279	21·008
7	33·708	29·651	28·458	27·598	26·980	26·545	26·069
8	40·641	35·856	34·415	33·347	32·548	31·947	31·172
9	47·885	42·308	40·578	39·258	38·229	37·416	36·257
10	55·412	48·962	46·896	45·274	43·969	42·898	41·282
11	63·191	55·775	53·322	51·350	49·722	48·356	46·228
12	71·193	62·706	59·815	57·445	55·456	53·762	51·088
13	79·389	69·721	66·341	63·531	61·146	59·103	55·865
14	87·749	76·789	72·873	69·585	66·780	64·372	60·566
15	96·247	83·881	79·387	75·592	72·349	69·568	65·203

'Singles' method (Li and Mantel, 1968). This is the simplest method of testing for recessive inheritance when there is complete ascertainment and according to the originators it is just as reliable as more involved methods. The method consists simply of determining the number of sibships in which there is only one affected individual (= 'singles') and

$$p = \frac{R - J}{T - J}$$

where

R = number of affected individuals in all sibships

T = total number of individuals in all sibships

J = number of 'singles'

Using the data as presented in Table 4.1 (p. 38).

$$p = \frac{19 - 4}{61 - 4}$$

$$= \frac{15}{57}$$

$$= 0 \cdot 263$$

Note the close agreement with the value obtained by the maximum likelihood method. Unfortunately though this is a very simple method for calculating 'p', the determination of the variance is complicated. Li and Mantel (1968) have shown that the variance is

$$\frac{1}{W}$$

where

$$W = \sum n_s w_s$$

where

$$w_s = \frac{s}{pq} \cdot \frac{(1 - q^{s-1})^2}{(1 - q^s)[1 - q^s + (s - 2)pq^{s-1}]}$$

Fortunately Li and Mantel (1968) have provided tables of 'w' for various 'p' values (Table 4.6). For example in the above example the following values of $w_s n_s$ are obtained:

Sibship size s	No. of sibships n_s	w_s	$w_s n_s$	
If $P = 0.26$				
2	1	3·43	3·43	
6	3	21·18	63·54	
7	2	26·49	52·98	
8	2	32·06	64·12	
11	1	49·72	49·72	$\therefore \sum w_s n_s = 233·79$
If $P = 0.27$				
2	1	3·39	3·39	
6	3	21·01	63·03	
7	2	26·29	52·58	
8	2	31·81	63·62	
11	1	49·18	49·18	$\therefore \sum w_s n_s = 231·80$

and by interpolation $\sum w_s n_s = 233·18$. Therefore the variance is $1/233·18$ and the standard error of the estimate is $1/\sqrt{233·18}$ or $0·065$.

Single incomplete ascertainment (Fisher, 1934)

The underlying assumption in this method (sometimes referred to as the 'sib' method) is that each affected individual has a very small chance of being ascertained, and therefore there is never more than one proband per family. The probability of ascertaining each family is proportional to the number of affected individuals in the family.

In this case

$$p = \frac{R - N}{T - N}$$

which has a variance of

$$\frac{pq}{T - N}$$

where

$R = $ number of affected individuals in all sibships

$T = $ total number of individuals in all sibships

$N = $ number of sibships

Table 4.6 'Singles' method of estimating the segregation ratio under complete ascertainment (*From* Li and Mantel, 1968)

Values of $w = \dfrac{s}{pq} \cdot \dfrac{(1 - q^{s-1})^2}{(1 - q^s)[1 - q^s + (s - 2)pq^{s-1}]}$

s	p = 0.16	p = 0.17	p = 0.18	p = 0.19	p = 0.20	p = 0.21	p = 0.22	p = 0.23	p = 0.24	p = 0.25
2	4.40	4.23	4.09	3.97	3.86	3.76	3.68	3.60	3.54	3.48
3	9.13	8.81	8.54	8.29	8.08	7.90	7.74	7.60	7.48	7.37
4	14.21	13.74	13.34	12.99	12.68	12.41	12.18	11.98	11.81	11.66
5	19.64	19.03	18.50	18.04	17.65	17.30	17.01	16.75	16.53	16.34
6	25.42	24.67	24.02	23.46	22.97	22.55	22.19	21.88	21.61	21.38
7	31.54	30.64	29.88	29.21	28.64	28.14	27.71	27.34	27.01	26.73
8	37.98	36.95	36.06	35.29	34.62	34.04	33.53	33.09	32.70	32.36
9	44.74	43.56	42.54	41.66	40.88	40.21	39.61	39.08	38.62	38.20
10	51.79	50.46	49.30	48.29	47.40	46.61	45.90	45.28	44.71	44.20
11	59.11	57.61	56.30	55.14	54.12	53.20	52.37	51.62	50.93	50.30
12	66.68	65.00	63.51	62.19	61.00	59.93	58.95	58.06	57.23	56.46
13	74.47	72.58	70.90	69.39	68.02	66.77	65.62	64.55	63.56	62.63
14	82.44	80.32	78.42	76.70	75.13	73.68	72.33	71.07	69.89	68.78
15	90.58	88.20	86.06	84.10	82.29	80.62	79.05	77.58	76.20	74.88
16	98.84	96.19	93.77	91.55	89.49	87.56	85.76	84.06	82.45	80.93
17	107.21	104.24	101.53	99.02	96.68	94.49	92.43	90.49	88.65	86.92
18	115.65	112.35	109.31	106.49	103.85	101.38	99.05	96.85	94.78	92.83
19	124.15	120.48	117.09	113.94	110.99	108.22	105.61	103.16	100.85	98.67
20	132.67	128.62	124.86	121.35	118.07	115.00	112.11	109.39	106.84	104.45

Table 4.6—continued

s	p = 0·25	p = 0·26	p = 0·27	p = 0·28	p = 0·29	p = 0·30	p = 0·31	p = 0·32	p = 0·33	p = 0·34
2	3·48	3·43	3·39	3·35	3·32	3·30	3·27	3·26	3·24	3·23
3	7·37	7·28	7·20	7·13	7·08	7·03	7·00	6·97	6·95	6·95
4	11·66	11·53	11·42	11·34	11·26	11·20	11·16	11·13	11·11	11·10
5	16·34	16·18	16·04	15·93	15·84	15·77	15·72	15·68	15·66	15·65
6	21·38	21·18	21·01	20·88	20·76	20·67	20·60	20·55	20·52	20·50
7	26·73	26·49	26·29	26·12	25·97	25·85	25·75	25·67	25·61	25·57
8	32·36	32·06	31·81	31·58	31·38	31·21	31·07	30·94	30·83	30·74
9	38·20	37·83	37·50	37·20	36·94	36·70	36·48	36·29	36·11	35·95
10	44·20	43·73	43·31	42·92	42·56	42·23	41·92	41·64	41·38	41·13
11	50·30	49·72	49·18	48·67	48·20	47·76	47·35	46·96	46·59	46·25
12	56·46	55·73	55·06	54·42	53·82	53·25	52·72	52·21	51·73	51·28
13	62·63	61·75	60·92	60·13	59·39	58·68	58·01	57·38	56·78	56·22
14	68·78	67·72	66·72	65·78	64·88	64·03	63·22	62·46	61·74	61·07
15	74·88	73·64	72·47	71·35	70·29	69·30	68·35	67·46	66·63	65·84
16	80·93	79·50	78·14	76·85	75·63	74·48	73·40	72·39	71·43	70·55
17	86·92	85·28	83·73	82·27	80·89	79·60	78·38	77·24	76·18	75·19
18	92·83	90·99	89·25	87·62	86·09	84·65	83·30	82·05	80·88	79·80
19	98·67	96·63	94·71	92·91	91·22	89·64	88·17	86·81	85·54	84·36
20	104·45	102·20	100·10	98·13	96·30	94·59	93·00	91·53	90·16	88·90

Table 4.6—*continued*

s	p = 0·05	p = 0·10	p = 0·15	p = 0·20	p = 0·25	p = 0·30	p = 0·35	p = 0·40	p = 0·45	p = 0·50
2	11·07	6·16	4·58	3·86	3·48	3·30	3·23	3·26	3·36	3·56
3	22·42	12·61	9·50	8·08	7·37	7·03	6·94	7·04	7·29	7·71
4	34·05	19·38	14·76	12·68	11·66	11·20	11·11	11·28	11·68	12·30
5	45·95	26·46	20·36	17·65	16·34	15·77	15·66	15·88	16·36	17·08
6	58·15	33·86	26·30	22·97	21·38	20·67	20·51	20·69	21·16	21·86
7	70·62	41·57	32·58	28·64	26·73	25·85	25·54	25·60	25·93	26·52
8	83·39	49·60	39·18	34·62	32·36	31·21	30·67	30·49	30·61	31·02
9	96·44	57·94	46·11	40·88	38·20	36·70	35·81	35·31	35·16	35·37
10	109·78	66·60	53·33	47·40	44·20	42·23	40·91	40·03	39·58	39·61
11	123·42	75·56	60·84	54·12	50·30	47·76	45·93	44·64	43·89	43·76
12	137·35	84·83	68·61	61·00	56·46	53·25	50·86	49·14	48·12	47·86
13	151·57	94·39	76·62	68·02	62·63	58·68	55·69	53·56	52·29	51·92
14	166·09	104·24	84·83	75·13	68·78	64·03	60·44	57·91	56·42	55·95
15	180·90	114·37	93·23	82·29	74·88	69·30	65·11	62·21	60·51	59·97
16	196·01	124·76	101·79	89·49	80·93	74·48	69·72	66·47	64·59	63·98
17	211·41	135·41	110·48	96·68	86·92	79·60	74·28	70·70	68·65	67·99
18	227·09	146·30	119·27	103·85	92·83	84·65	78·79	74·91	72·70	71·99
19	243·08	157·41	128·15	110·99	98·67	89·64	83·28	79·11	76·75	76·00
20	259·35	168·73	137·08	118·07	104·45	94·59	87·74	83·29	80·80	80·00

Table 4.6—continued

s	$p = 0.50$	$p = 0.55$	$p = 0.60$	$p = 0.65$	$p = 0.70$	$p = 0.75$	$p = 0.80$	$p = 0.85$	$p = 0.90$	$p = 0.95$
2	3·56	3·84	4·25	4·82	5·64	6·83	8·68	11·86	18·37	38·19
3	7·71	8·31	9·13	10·23	11·74	13·85	17·01	22·21	32·44	62·71
4	12·30	13·14	14·26	15·71	17·66	20·36	24·37	31·01	44·28	84·17
5	17·08	18·04	19·29	20·93	23·14	26·28	31·05	39·13	55·53	105·26
6	21·86	22·81	24·10	25·84	28·28	31·86	37·44	47·04	66·66	126·32
7	26·52	27·40	28·67	30·51	33·21	37·29	43·73	54·90	77·78	147·37
8	31·02	31·80	33·07	35·05	38·05	42·65	50·00	62·74	88·89	168·42
9	35·37	36·06	37·37	39·51	42·84	48·00	56·25	70·59	100·00	189·47
10	39·61	40·24	41·60	43·93	47·61	53·33	62·50	78·43	111·11	210·53
11	43·76	44·35	45·80	48·34	52·38	58·67	68·75	86·27	122·22	231·58
12	47·86	48·44	49·98	52·74	57·14	64·00	75·00	94·12	133·33	252·63
13	51·92	52·50	54·16	57·14	61·90	69·33	81·25	101·96	144·44	273·68
14	55·95	56·55	58·33	61·54	66·67	74·67	87·50	109·80	155·56	294·74
15	59·97	60·60	62·50	65·93	71·43	80·00	93·75	117·65	166·67	315·79
16	63·98	64·64	66·67	70·33	76·19	85·33	100·00	125·49	177·78	336·84
17	67·99	68·68	70·83	74·73	80·95	90·67	106·25	133·33	188·89	357·89
18	71·99	72·73	75·00	79·12	85·71	96·00	112·50	141·18	200·00	378·95
19	76·00	76·77	79·17	83·52	90·48	101·33	118·75	149·02	211·11	400·00
20	80·00	80·81	83·33	87·91	95·24	106·67	125·00	156·86	222·22	421·05

If we apply this approach to the data in Table 4.1 (p. 38) then

$$p = \frac{19 - 9}{61 - 9}$$

$$= \frac{10}{52}$$

$$= 0 \cdot 192$$

and the standard error of this estimate is

$$\sqrt{\frac{pq}{T - N}}$$

$$= \sqrt{\frac{(0 \cdot 192)(0 \cdot 808)}{52}}$$

$$= 0 \cdot 055$$

The estimate of 'p' calculated in this way would therefore appear to be less than expected. When inappropriately applied this method in fact tends to underestimate the value of 'p'. However in this example the value obtained has wide 95 per cent confidence limits because the numbers are small (i.e. $0 \cdot 192 \pm (1 \cdot 96)(0 \cdot 055)$ or $0 \cdot 084$ to $0 \cdot 300$), which would accommodate a theoretical value for 'p' of $0 \cdot 25$.

Multiple incomplete ascertainment (Bailey, 1951; Morton, 1959)

In practice, ascertainment varies being somewhere between complete and single incomplete in which case the method of multiple incomplete ascertainment is the most appropriate for analysis, particularly of families who present to the clinician. There is often more than one proband per sibship but not all affected individuals are probands. Under such circumstances the simplest method of determining the proportion of affected sibs of probands is to count each sibship once for each time it has been independently ascertained, omitting the proband each time. This is sometimes referred to as Weinberg's 'proband' method.

The method is illustrated in data from a random sample of families with phenylketonuria (Table 4.7).

In this case

$$p = \frac{8}{32}$$

$$= 0 \cdot 25$$

More refined statistical methods for analysing family data under multiple incomplete ascertainment are available but they are complex and are beyond the scope of this book. In any event there is no universal agreement as to their assumptions and statistical validity.

Table 4.7 Analysis of family data assuming multiple incomplete ascertainment. The proband in each sibship is indicated by an arrow (normal: male □, female ○ ; affected: male ■, female ●).

Family	Number in sibship		
	Probands	Affected sibs.	Total sibs.
1 ■ ○ ○ ○	1	0	3
2 ○ ● ●	1	1	2
3 □ ○ ■	1	0	2
4 □ ● □ ■ □	1	1	4
5 ■ ● ○ □ ○	2	$\begin{cases} 1 \\ 1 \end{cases}$	4 4
6 ■ ●	1	1	1
7 □ ● □ ● ○	1	1	4
8 ● ○ ○ □	1	0	3
9 ■ ○	1	0	1
10 ■ ○ ■	2	$\begin{cases} 1 \\ 1 \end{cases}$	2 2
Total		8	32

In conclusion, in analysing family data where one may not be entirely certain of the precise mode of ascertainment and which affected individuals are probands and which are secondary cases, an approximate value of 'p' can be obtained in the following way. The frequency among sibs is calculated assuming complete ascertainment which will tend to give an *over* estimate. The value is then calculated assuming single incomplete ascertainment which will tend to give an *under* estimate. The true value will be somewhere between these two extremes or, more precisely, between the two most extreme confidence limits derived from the two methods.

X-Linked inheritance

In X-linked inheritance (whether dominant or recessive) for rare disorders there is never male to male transmission. Simple pedigree inspection may therefore exclude the possibility of X-linked inheritance.

In X-linked *dominant* inheritance, if fully penetrant, *all* the daughters of affected males will be affected. In the case of affected females, on average, half their daughters and half their sons will be affected. A departure from the expected 1:1 ratio of affected to normal offspring of affected females may be tested for in the same way as for auto-somal dominant inheritance (p. 35).

In X-linked *recessive* inheritance *all* the daughters of affected males will be carriers. In the case of carrier females, on average, half their daughters will also be carriers and half their sons will be affected. A departure from the expected 1:1 ratio of affected to normal sons of *known* carriers may be tested for as in the case of autosomal dominant inheritance provided the selection of carriers was because they were the daughters of affected males. If they have been selected in any other way this introduces biases into the calculations which would have to be taken into account, for example if carriers have been selected because they have had at least one affected son and also another affected maternal male relative. In this situation one might apply the method of multiple incomplete ascertainment to the male progeny of such carriers.

In serious disorders where affected males are infertile or do not survive to have children it may be very difficult to prove X-linkage. However there are statistical methods, though somewhat complex, for getting round this problem (Morton and Chung, 1959). Otherwise one may have to resort to evidence other than segregation analysis, for example, the same woman may have had affected sons by more than one father, though this does not exclude autosomal dominant inheritance with male limitation. The best proof is the demonstration of linkage with an X-linked marker trait such as the Xg blood group, glucose-6-phosphate dehydrogenase deficiency or colour blindness.

5. Multifactorial Inheritance

In many common disorders (e.g. diabetes mellitus, schizophrenia, peptic ulcer and hypertension) and a number of congenital malformations (e.g. spina bifida and anencephaly, congenital pyloric stenosis and congenital dislocation of the hip) there is a definite familial tendency, the proportion of affected relatives being greater than in the general population but the proportion of affected relatives is often only of the order of 5 per cent or less, and therefore much less than would be expected on a simple unifactorial basis. The most likely explanation is that these disorders are inherited on a *multifactorial* basis. This implies that the cause is partly environmental and partly due to the effects of many genes each of small effect.

If the observed familial aggregation in a particular disorder is suspected of being the result of multifactorial inheritance this may be tested for in a number of ways. It must always be remembered, however, that a confounding feature will be if there is genetic heterogeneity in the disorder being studied. This possibility must be carefully considered and, as far as possible, excluded before combining data from different individuals and their families.

Tests for multifactorial inheritance

A number of models have been proposed for multifactorial inheritance but the one which is most widely used is referred to as the 'threshold model' (Falconer, 1965). According to this model it is assumed that there is some underlying graded attribute which is related to the causation of a particular disorder or congenital malformation. This is referred to as the individual's *liability* which includes not only his genetic predisposition but also the environmental circumstances which render him more or less likely to develop the disease. According to the model the curve of liability has a normal distribution in both the general population and relatives of probands but the curve for relatives is shifted to the right because they have a higher mean liability (Fig. 5.1). The point on the curve beyond which all individuals are affected is the *threshold*. In the general population the proportion above the threshold is the population frequency and among relatives the proportion above the threshold is the familial frequency.

There are several consequences of such a model and if these are demonstrable in a particular family study it indicates that the disorder in question is probably inherited on a multifactorial basis.

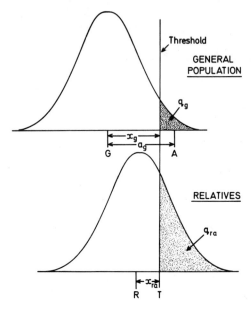

Fig. 5.1 Hypothetical curves of liability in the general population and in relatives of probands.

1. The fall off in frequency from first-degree to second-degree to third-degree relatives can be predicted from the threshold model and will be greater than that predicted on the basis of unifactorial inheritance. Examples of this phenomenon have been given by Carter (1976).

2. The frequency will be greatest among the relatives of more severely affected individuals because presumably they are more extreme deviants along the curve of liability.

3. The frequency among sibs born subsequent to index cases will be greater the more affected relatives there are in a family, presumably because this indicates that there are more abnormal genes segregating in the family and/or the family has been more exposed to a precipitating environmental factor(s).

4. When there is a sex difference in the population frequency, the frequency among relatives of affected individuals of the less frequently affected sex will be greater than the frequency among relatives of affected individuals of the more frequently affected sex. This is presumably because affected individuals of the less frequently affected sex will tend to be more extreme deviants from the population mean and so the risk to their relatives will be correspondingly higher.

Other expectations of multifactorial inheritance, though *not* directly consequent on the threshold model, are:

5. The *frequency* among first-degree relatives is approximately equal

to $\sqrt{q}$ where 'q' is the frequency in the general population (Edwards, 1960). Note that it is customary in discussing multifactorial inheritance for q to denote the frequency of the disorder and not gene frequency.

6. The *relative frequency* (referred to as 'K' by Penrose, 1953) is, for each sex, the frequency in relatives divided by the frequency in the general population. The observed relative frequencies can be compared with the expected values for various modes of inheritance.

Thus the expected relative frequencies in *sibs* are:

$$\frac{1}{2q} \quad \text{for an autosomal dominant trait}$$

$$\frac{1}{4q} \quad \text{for an autosomal recessive trait}$$

$$\frac{1}{\sqrt{q}} \quad \text{for a multifactorial trait.}$$

Thus in one study of sacro-iliitis (a manifestation of ankylosing spondylitis) the results in Table 5.1 were obtained. The fairly close agreement between the observed relative frequencies and those expected for multifactorial inheritance suggests that this disorder is inherited on this basis.

Table 5.1 Frequencies and relative frequencies of sacro-iliitis in sibs (data from Emery and Lawrence, 1967)

	Frequency		Observed	Relative frequency Expected		
	Gen. pop. (q)	Sibs. (s)	(s/q)	Dominant ($1/2q$)	Recessive ($1/4q$)	Multi-factorial ($1/\sqrt{q}$)
Males	0·04918	0·1585	3·22	10·17	5·08	4·51
Females	0·01515	0·1666	10·99	33·00	16·50	8·12

Estimation of heritability from family studies

Having decided that the disorder in question appears to be inherited on a multifactorial basis, it is useful to estimate the heritability. This may be defined as the proportion of the total phenotypic variance (genetic and nongenetic) which is due to additive genetic variance. It is therefore expressed as a percentage and abbreviated to the symbol 'h^2'. The greater the value for the heritability the greater the contribution of genetic factors to aetiology. There are, however, some important precautions to be borne in mind in estimating the heritability.

The estimation of heritability is only meaningful if there is no genetic heterogeneity in the disorder being studied and if no major gene contributes to the causation of the disorder. If a dominant gene contributes significantly to aetiology then the estimated heritability may exceed 100 per cent. If a recessive gene contributes significantly to aetiology then the estimated heritability from sibs will be much higher than that from parents and children. If, therefore, a 'reasonable' estimate of heritability is obtained, and this is roughly the same for sibs as for parents and children, then it would seem likely that the disorder in question is inherited on a multifactorial basis. Some estimates of heritability are given in Table 5.2.

Table 5.2 Estimates of heritability for various disorders affecting man

Disorder	Frequency (%)	Heritability
Schizophrenia	1	85
Asthma	4	80
Cleft lip ± cleft palate	0·1	76
Pyloric stenosis (congenital)	0·3	75
Diabetes mellitus: early onset	0·2	75
late onset	2–3	35
Ankylosing spondylitis	0·2	70
Club foot (congenital)	0·1	68
Coronary artery disease	3	65
Hypertension (essential)	5	62
Dislocation of the hip (congenital)	0·1	60
Anencephaly and spina bifida	0·5	60
Peptic ulcer	4	37
Congenital heart disease (all types)	0·5	35

In estimating heritability there are two important possible sources of error. Firstly, since heritability is estimated from the degree of resemblance between relatives, expressed as a correlation coefficient, a sharing of common environment by family members may result in the estimate being too high due to non-genetic causes of resemblance between relatives. This error is likely to affect sibs more than other relatives. For this reason it is therefore important to derive estimates from different kinds of relatives and to measure the frequency in relatives reared or living apart and in unrelated individuals living together, such as spouses. In this way it may be possible to assess the contribution from shared environmental factors. The second source of error only occurs when estimates are based on full sibs. This is due to the fact that non-additive genetic variance contributes to correlations between full sibs. For these two reasons heritability estimates should ideally be based not only on sibs but also on parents and offspring and, where possible, on second- and third-degree relatives though clearly this is usually a counsel of perfection.

Finally, in estimating heritability it is assumed that the variance of liability is the same in all groups being compared. It is therefore important that the 'general population' should be representative of the population from which affected individuals and their relatives are selected.

Calculation of heritability

In practice, the most usual situation is that in which the frequency of the disorder has been estimated in the general population ('g') and in relatives of affected individuals ('ra') (Method I in Falconer, 1965).

If A = affected individuals in a sample
   N = total number of individuals in the sample
   q = frequency = A/N
   $p = 1 - q$
   x = deviation of the threshold from the mean of the population
   a = deviation of the mean of affecteds from the mean of the population
   r = correlation between relatives and probands.
   V = sampling variance of r

$$W = \frac{p}{a^2 A}$$

then
$$r = \frac{x_g - x_{ra}}{a_g}$$

and $h^2 = r$ for identical (MZ) twins
      $= 2r$ for first-degree relatives and non-identical (DZ) twins
      $= 4r$ for second-degree relatives
      $= 8r$ for third-degree relatives.

That is $h^2 = r/R$ where 'R' is the coefficient of relationship (see p. 20).

From tables of the normal distribution, given a frequency 'q', it is possible to determine the normal deviate 'x' (single-tailed), in standard deviation units, of the threshold from the population mean and also 'a' the deviation of the mean of the affecteds from the population mean (Appendix 5, p. 136). If the frequency in the general population is assumed to have been estimated without serious error (*see* Falconer, 1965) then the variance can be calculated thus:

$$V \simeq \left(\frac{1}{a}\right)_g^2 W_{ra}$$

and
$$\text{s.e. } h^2 = 2\sqrt{V} \quad \text{for first-degree relatives}$$
$$= 4\sqrt{V} \quad \text{for second-degree relatives}$$
$$= 8\sqrt{V} \quad \text{for third-degree relatives}$$

If the frequency of a disorder differs in the two sexes, then the sexes of both probands and relatives must be treated separately giving four estimates of heritability: male relatives of male probands, female relatives of male probands, male relatives of female probands and female relatives of female probands. Here we have three frequencies: general population comparable to affected individuals ('g'), general population comparable with relatives ('gr') and relatives of affected individuals ('ra'). In this situation

$$r = \frac{x_{gr} - x_{ra}}{a_g}$$

and
$$V \simeq \left(\frac{1}{a}\right)_g^2 (W_{gr} + W_{ra})$$

If the four separate estimates of the heritability do not differ significantly they can be combined into a single estimate by weighting each by the reciprocal of its sampling variance and taking a weighted mean.

Another situation is when the data consist of the frequencies in relatives of affected individuals ('ra') and in relatives of unaffected controls matched for age and sex with the affected individuals ('c'). In this situation

$$r = \frac{p_c(x_c - x_{ra})}{a_c}$$

and
$$V \simeq \left(\frac{p}{a}\right)_c^2 W_{ra}$$

Worked examples involving these various methods are given by Falconer (1965) and also the special case in which there is variable age of onset (Falconer, 1967). The reader can be no better advised than to refer to the original publications. However, a simple example may perhaps be helpful in illustrating the method of calculation.

Wynne-Davies (1970) has made a study of the frequency of congenital dislocation of the hip in various relatives of affected individuals. If we use the data on so-called 'late-diagnosis' cases the population frequency is about one per 1000, i.e. $q_g = 0.1$ per cent. From Appendix 5 for $q_g = 0.1$ per cent, values for x_g and a_g are 3.090 and 3.367. Among first-degree relatives there were 35 affected individuals out of 1777, i.e. $q_{ra} = 1.97$ per cent. From Appendix 5 for $q_{ra} = 1.97$ per cent, values for x_{ra} and a_{ra} are 2.060 and 2.426.

Since

$$r = \frac{x_g - x_{ra}}{a_g}$$

therefore
$$r = \frac{3\cdot090 - 2\cdot060}{3\cdot367}$$
$$= 0\cdot306$$

$$h^2 = 2r \text{ for first-degree relatives}$$

therefore $\quad h^2 = 61\cdot2$ per cent

Now
$$V = \left(\frac{1}{a}\right)_g^2 W_{ra}$$

$$= \left(\frac{1}{a}\right)_g^2 \left(\frac{p}{a^2 A}\right)_{ra}$$

$$= \left(\frac{1}{3\cdot367}\right)^2 \left(\frac{0\cdot9803}{(2\cdot426)^2 35}\right)$$

$$= 0\cdot000420$$

s.e. $h^2 = 2\sqrt{V}$ for first-degree relatives

therefore $\quad$ s.e. $h^2 = 0\cdot041$

or $\quad\quad\quad\quad\quad\quad\quad\quad 4\cdot1$ per cent

Similarly the heritability and the standard error can be calculated for second- and third-degree relatives (Table 5.3), the estimates obtained being $45\cdot6 \pm 9\cdot8$ and $46\cdot4 \pm 26\cdot3$.

In these calculations it has been assumed that the frequency in the general population (0·10 per cent) is known without error, i.e. that the number of affecteds upon which q_g was estimated was very large. This of course simplifies the situation but tends to reduce the estimated standard errors slightly.

The three estimates of the heritability can be combined by weighting each by the reciprocal of its sampling variance and taking a weighted mean, i.e. by dividing each of the individual heritability estimates by its variance and summing, and dividing this by the sum of the reciprocals of the variances. Thus

$$\text{weighted mean of } h^2 = \frac{\dfrac{h_1^2}{(\text{s.e.}_1)^2} + \dfrac{h_2^2}{(\text{s.e.}_2)^2} + \dfrac{h_3^2}{(\text{s.e.}_3)^2}}{\dfrac{1}{(\text{s.e.}_1)^2} + \dfrac{1}{(\text{s.e.}_2)^2} + \dfrac{1}{(\text{s.e.}_3)^2}}$$

$$= \frac{\dfrac{61\cdot2}{(4\cdot1)^2} + \dfrac{45\cdot6}{(9\cdot8)^2} + \dfrac{46\cdot4}{(26\cdot3)^2}}{\dfrac{1}{(4\cdot1)^2} + \dfrac{1}{(9\cdot8)^2} + \dfrac{1}{(26\cdot3)^2}}$$

$$= 58\cdot6 \text{ per cent}$$

The sampling variance of this combined estimate is approximately the reciprocal of the sum of the weights. Thus

$$\text{s.e. of the weighted mean} = \frac{1}{\sqrt{\dfrac{1}{(\text{s.e.}_1)^2} + \dfrac{1}{(\text{s.e.}_2)^2} + \dfrac{1}{(\text{s.e.}_3)^2}}}$$

$$= \frac{1}{\sqrt{\dfrac{1}{(4 \cdot 1)^2} + \dfrac{1}{(9 \cdot 8)^2} + \dfrac{1}{(26 \cdot 3)^2}}}$$

$$= 3 \cdot 7 \text{ per cent}$$

Thus the combined estimate of the heritability with its standard error is $58 \cdot 6 \pm 3 \cdot 7$ per cent.

Table 5.3 Heritability of congenital dislocation of the hip (late diagnosis) from frequencies in various relatives (data from Wynne-Davies, 1970)

	A	N	$q\%$	x	a	r	$V \times 1000$	$\sqrt{V}$	$h^2 \pm$ s.e.
Population	—	—	0·10	3·090	3·367	—	—	—	—
Relatives:									
first-degree	35	1777	1·97	2·060	2·426	0·306	0·420	0·0205	61·2 ± 4·1
second-degree	16	4746	0·34	2·706	3·012	0·114	0·606	0·0246	45·6 ± 9·8
third-degree	8	4220	0·19	2·894	3·185	0·058	1·085	0·0329	46·4 ± 26·3

Not all investigators agree with Falconer's model and consider that it is perhaps somewhat artificial to imagine a sharp cut-off beyond which individuals are affected. Instead Edwards (1969) and Curnow (1972) have suggested that a more realistic model is to consider that the genetic component of liability is normally distributed in both the general population and in affected individuals and according to Curnow (1972) the risk of being affected increases in a sigmoid manner from 0 at a low genetic level to 1 at a high genetic level. However, Falconer's model and this latter model are mathematically equivalent and lead to similar results.

Smith (1970) has produced a very useful graph (Fig. 5.2) from which it is possible to derive an approximate estimate of the correlation in liability between relatives, knowing the frequency of a disorder in the general population and in relatives of affected individuals. Knowing the correlation coefficient (r) it is possible to calculate the heritability since $h^2 = r/R$ where 'R' is the coefficient of relationship (see p. 20). Thus in the case of renal calculi (an example chosen by Falconer, 1965) the frequency in relatives of controls is 0·4 per cent and the frequency in first-degree relatives of patients is 2·5 per cent. From Smith's graph

$r = 0.25$ and therefore the heritability is 50 per cent. From Figure 5.2 it is also possible to estimate the standard error of the heritability (Smith, 1970), but the method is complex and it is easier to calculate using Falconer's method (Falconer, 1965) as illustrated on p. 55. Note that because of sampling error the frequency in relatives might, in a particular study, appear to be less than the population frequency which would give rise to a negative estimate of heritability (Fig. 5.2). Such negative estimates should be included when pooling estimates from different sources.

Provided the population frequency of a disorder is known it is also possible from Smith's graph (Fig. 5.2) to derive an approximate estimate of the *upper limit* of recurrence risks for relatives by assuming h^2 is 100 per cent. Thus if the frequency in the general population is 1.0 per cent the maximum frequency (recurrence risk) among first-degree relatives $(r = 0.5)$ is 13 per cent, among second-degree relatives $(r = 0.25)$ is 4.5 per cent and among third-degree relatives $(r = 0.125)$ is about 2.2 per cent. The values obtained by Falconer's method are very similar and from the practical point of view of genetic counselling the differences are small enough to be ignored.

So far we have only been concerned with the estimation of heritability of *discontinuous* characters. Prominence has been given to this subject because most disease states are regarded in this way. However mention should also be made of the estimation of heritability of *continuous* characters such as stature and blood pressure. Here heritability is estimated either from parent–offspring correlations or sib–sib correlations. In the former we take the average value of the offspring in each family and then calculate the correlation (r) between these values and the average value for both parents in each family (so-called *mid-parent* value), in which case

$$h^2 = \frac{r}{0.71}$$

or calculate the correlation (r) between the average values of the offspring in each family and the value for *one* parent in each family (the mother–child and father–child correlations being treated separately), in which case

$$h^2 = 2r$$

In the case of sibs one calculates the so-called intraclass correlation coefficient by an analysis of variance. The reader is referred to one of the standard text books of statistics for details which are outside the scope of this book (for example, see Snedecor and Cochran, 1967, p. 294 *et seq.*). The derivation of heritability from the intraclass correlation for sibs is not straightforward and the problem is discussed by Falconer (Falconer, 1960).

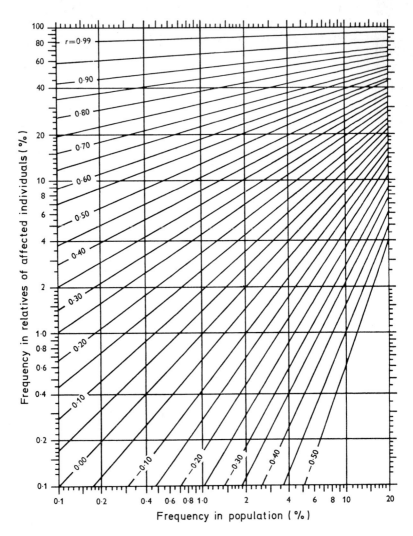

Fig. 5.2 Graph of correlations in liability (r) between relatives and probands. From this the heritability (h^2) can be derived since $h^2 = r$ for MZ twins, $h^2 = 2r$ for first-degree relatives, $h^2 = 4r$ for second-degree relatives and $h^2 = 8r$ for third-degree relatives. (From Smith, 1970.)

Estimation of heritability from twin studies

Twins are said to be *concordant* when both exhibit the same trait. If only one twin has the trait they are said to be discordant (see p. 84).

If in a particular disorder the population frequency and the proband concordance rate (C_n) in twins are known then it is possible to estimate the correlation ('r') in liability and from this the heritability (Smith, 1974). An estimate of 'r' is given by

$$r = \frac{x_g - x_{ra}}{a_g}$$

where values of 'x' and 'a' can be obtained from Appendix 5 in the usual manner. Thus if the frequency of a disorder in the population is 0·5 per cent ($x_g = 2\cdot576$ and $a_g = 2\cdot892$) and if the proband concordance rate is 5·0 per cent ($x_{ra} = 1\cdot645$) then

$$r = \frac{2\cdot576 - 1\cdot645}{2\cdot892}$$

$$= 0\cdot32$$

or a more precise estimate may be obtained from

$$r = \frac{x_g - [x_{ra}\sqrt{1 - (x_g^2 - x_{ra}^2)(1 - x_g/a_g)}]}{a_g + [x_{ra}^2(a_g - x_g)]}$$

which in the above example is

$$= \frac{2\cdot576 - [1\cdot645\sqrt{1 - (2\cdot576^2 - 1\cdot645^2)(1 - 2\cdot576/2\cdot892)}]}{2\cdot892 + [1\cdot645^2(2\cdot892 - 2\cdot576)]}$$

$$= 0\cdot36$$

The standard error of the correlation

$$\text{s.e.} = \sqrt{\left(\frac{1}{a_g^2}\right)\left(\frac{1}{a_{ra}^2}\right)\left(\frac{1 - C_p}{A}\right)}$$

Where A in this case is the number of twin pairs in which both members are affected. Thus, if in the above example $A = 9$ then

$$\text{s.e.} = \sqrt{\left(\frac{1}{2\cdot892^2}\right)\left(\frac{1}{2\cdot063^2}\right)\left(\frac{0\cdot95}{9}\right)}$$

$$= 0\cdot05$$

Thus the estimate of the correlation and its standard error in the above example is

$$0\cdot36 \pm 0\cdot05$$

It is also possible from twin data to estimate the correlation and therefore the heritability simply from Figure 5.2, provided the concordance rate in twins and the frequency in the population are known. Thus in schizophrenia the population frequency is about 1·0 per cent and in one recent study the proband concordance rates were approximately 58 per cent in MZ twins and 12 per cent in DZ twins

(Gottesman and Shields, 1972, see p. 84). From Figure 5.2 if the concordance in MZ twins is 58 per cent then r_{MZ} is 0·92, and if concordance in DZ twins is 12 per cent then r_{DZ} is 0·48. Therefore for MZ twins

$$h^2 = r_{MZ} = 92 \text{ per cent}$$

and for DZ twins

$$h^2 = 2r_{DZ} = 96 \text{ per cent}$$

Pooling the results of several such twin studies the average estimate of the heritability of schizophrenia works out to be about 85 per cent (Gottesman and Shields, 1973).

It should be noted that in the absence of environmental similarities, concordance rates in MZ twins will not be expected to be high unless the heritability and population frequencies are high (Smith, 1970). Despite a high heritability the concordance may be low if the population frequency is low.

It should also be noted that the index (H) proposed by Holzinger (Holzinger, 1929), which depends on concordance rates in MZ and DZ twins (i.e. $H = (C_{MZ} - C_{DZ})/(1 - C_{DZ})$), is an arbitrary index and has no specific genetic interpretation (p. 88). It is not a measure of heritability and therefore should not be used for this purpose (Smith, 1974).

The heritability of *continuous* characters may also be estimated from twin studies, in this case it is derived from the intraclass correlation coefficient and this is discussed later (p. 87).

In conclusion, an estimate of heritability of liability for a particular disorder is valuable for a number of reasons. Firstly, if a 'reasonable' estimate is obtained this tends to support the hypothesis that the disorder is inherited on a multifactorial basis. Secondly, it gives an idea of the relative contribution of genetic and environmental factors to aetiology. Thirdly, it can be useful in genetic counselling in helping to predict the possible frequency (and therefore the chances of recurrence) in relatives.

6. Genetic Linkage

Recently the study of human-animal hybrid cells has provided a great deal of information on gene localization in man. Pedigree analysis, however, will continue to be of value particularly for localizing genes for traits not expressed in cultured cells and for measuring distances between loci.

Much has been written on the subject of pedigree analysis for genetic linkage studies and detailed expositions are to be found in some recent publications (Edwards, 1971; Renwick, 1971; Smith, 1968). An eminently readable introduction to the subject is to be found in Race and Sanger's book *Blood Groups in Man* (Race and Sanger, 1975).

The method adopted in determining linkage is the maximum likelihood estimate of the recombination fraction (usually referred to as θ) based upon the relative probability (P_R) of having obtained the family. The latter is determined by calculating the probability of having obtained the various combinations of the particular traits under consideration on the assumption of there being no measurable linkage $(\theta = 0 \cdot 5)$ and comparing this with the probabilities based on a range of recombination fractions from $0 \cdot 00$ to $0 \cdot 50$, i.e.

$$P_R = \frac{P \text{ (family, given } \theta = 0 \text{ to } 0 \cdot 5)}{P \text{ (family, given } \theta = 0 \cdot 5)}$$

For convenience P_R is often expressed as its logarithm. The $\log_{10}$ of the relative probability is called the log of the odds or the *lod score*. The maximum likelihood estimate of θ may be obtained by plotting the sum of the lod scores (or the relative probabilities) for all the families studied against various values of θ from $0 \cdot 00$ to $0 \cdot 50$, and is the value of θ corresponding to the peak of the curve.

Autosomal linkage

Three generation families

Linkage phase refers to whether two linked genes are on the same particular chromosome (= *coupling phase*) or on different homologous chromosomes (= *repulsion phase*). In three generation families the linkage phase of individuals in the second generation may be obvious from inspection of the pedigree. In such a situation the recombination fraction can be determined quite simply. Thus in the family in Figure 6.1, if black represents myotonic dystrophy, a dominant disorder, and the secretor alleles are represented as *Se* (secretor) which is dominant to *se* (non-secretor) for the presence of ABH substances in body secretions, we see that II_1 must be heterozygous for both loci, and the secretor and myotonic genes are in coupling in II_1. Therefore in the third generation III_{2-6} are all non-recombinants but III_1 is a recombinant.

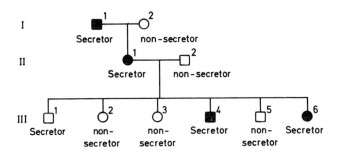

Fig. 6.1 Family in which myotonic dystrophy (dominant) and secretor status are segregating.

In this situation the recombination fraction (θ) is therefore 1 out of 6 or 0·17. In fact, the study of a large number of families in which secretor status and myotonic dystrophy were segregating gives a value of θ close to 0·07.

Two generation families

When information is available only in two generations of a family, the measurement of linkage is more involved and demands a resort to some mathematics. If '*G*' and '*g*' are alleles at the 'main' (disease) locus and '*T*' and '*t*' are alleles at the 'test' (genetic marker) locus, then if an individual has the genotype *GT/gt* (i.e. coupling phase) there are four possible types of gametes: two non-recombinants (*GT* and *gt*) and two recombinants (*Gt* and *gT*). If the frequency of recombination is θ then:

$$\text{frequency of non-recombinant gametes} = 1 - \theta$$

$$\text{therefore frequency of } GT \text{ or } gt \text{ gametes} = \frac{1 - \theta}{2}$$

$$\text{and frequency of recombinant gametes} = \theta$$

$$\text{therefore frequency of } Gt \text{ or } gT \text{ gametes} = \frac{\theta}{2}$$

If these two loci were not on the same chromosome pair, or if linked were far apart, then there would be equal numbers of all four types of gametes.

Now let us consider a family in which Lutheran blood groups and secretor status are segregating. The Lutheran alleles are Lu^a and Lu^b where Lu^a is dominant to Lu^b (Fig. 6.2).

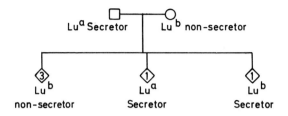

Fig. 6.2 Segregation of Lutheran blood groups and secretor status.

From this pedigree the mother must have the genotype Lu^bse/Lu^bse and father must be Lu^aSe/Lu^bse or Lu^aSe/Lu^bSe. Depending on which genotype the father has affects the assessment of his offspring as to which are recombinants and which are not. Let us first consider that the arrangement is Lu^aSe/Lu^bse, in which case the first four children are all non-recombinants and the last child is a recombinant (Fig. 6.3).

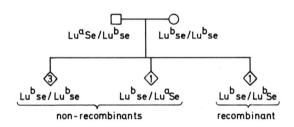

Fig. 6.3 Segregation of Lutheran blood groups and secretor status.

In this case the probability of getting

$$3 \text{ children} \quad Lu^bse/Lu^bse = \left(\frac{1-\theta}{2}\right)^3$$

$$1 \text{ child} \quad Lu^bse/Lu^aSe = \frac{1-\theta}{2}$$

$$1 \text{ child} \quad Lu^bse/Lu^bSe = \frac{\theta}{2}$$

Therefore the probability of getting this family if father has the genotype Lu^aSe/Lu^bse is

$$\left(\frac{1-\theta}{2}\right)^3\left(\frac{1-\theta}{2}\right)\left(\frac{\theta}{2}\right)$$

$$=\frac{\theta(1-\theta)^4}{32}$$

Now let us consider the alternative possibilities when the father has the genotype Lu^ase/Lu^bSe. Here the first four children are now all recombinants and the last child is a non-recombinant (Fig. 6.4).

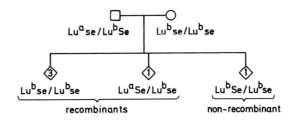

Fig. 6.4 Segregation of Lutheran blood groups and secretor status.

In this case the probability of getting

$$3 \text{ children} \quad Lu^bse/Lu^bse = \left(\frac{\theta}{2}\right)^3$$

$$1 \text{ child} \quad Lu^aSe/Lu^bse = \frac{\theta}{2}$$

$$1 \text{ child} \quad Lu^bSe/Lu^bse = \frac{1-\theta}{2}$$

Therefore the probability of getting this family if father has the genotype Lu^ase/Lu^bSe is

$$\left(\frac{\theta}{2}\right)^3\left(\frac{\theta}{2}\right)\left(\frac{1-\theta}{2}\right)$$

$$=\frac{\theta^4(1-\theta)}{32}$$

Now what we have to decide is the probability of obtaining the observed phenotypes of the children under two different assumptions namely that father is either in coupling or in repulsion. Since coupling and repulsion are equally likely the probability of getting this family is the *average* of the probabilities assuming coupling and repulsion, i.e.

$$\frac{1}{2}\left[\frac{\theta(1-\theta)^4}{32}+\frac{\theta^4(1-\theta)}{32}\right]$$

If we assume $\theta = 0.2$ then

$$P_{0.2} = \frac{1}{2}\left[\frac{(0.2)(0.8)^4}{32}+\frac{(0.2)^4(0.8)}{32}\right]$$

$$= 0.001300$$

If $\theta = 0.5$ then

$$P_{0.5} = \frac{1}{2}\left[\frac{(0.5)^5}{16}\right]$$

$$= 0.000976$$

Therefore the relative probability (P_R) when $\theta = 0.2$

$$= \frac{P\ (\text{family}\,|\,\theta = 0.2)}{P\ (\text{family}\,|\,\theta = 0.5)}\;*$$

$$= \frac{0.001300}{0.000976}$$

$$= 1.3320$$

This is then repeated for various values of θ from 0·0 to 0·5 (Table 6.1).

Table 6.1 Lutheran blood groups and secretor status: relative probabilities and lod scores

	Recombination fractions (θ)					
	0·0	0·1	0·2	0·3	0·4	0·5
Relative probability	0·0	1·0517	1·3320	1·2439	1·0758	1·0000
Lod score	$-\alpha$	0·022	0·124	0·095	0·031	0·00

The relative probabilities are then plotted against the various recombination fractions and in this way the maximum likelihood estimate of the recombination fraction is obtained (Fig. 6.5). In this example the maximum likelihood estimate of θ is approximately 0·23. In fact the study of a number of families in which the Lutheran blood groups and secretor status were segregating indicates that θ is about 0·15.

---

* 'P (family$|\theta = 0.2$)' means the probability of the family *given that* $\theta = 0.2$. The vertical line means 'given that'.

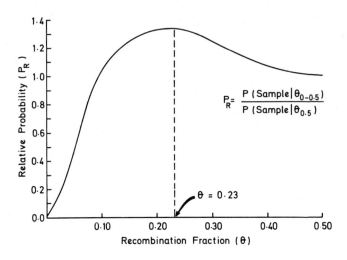

Fig. 6.5 Relative probability of linkage for various recombination fractions.

Fortunately it is not necessary to go through such laborious calculations each time because tables of lod scores are now available. The lod scores in Appendix 6 (p. 141) have been calculated from Smith, C. A. B. (1968) with some additional values specially made available by Professor C. A. B. Smith, and the table is presented in the convenient form adopted by Race and Sanger (1975).

When the parents' 'phase' is known (as it may be in three generation families) then lod scores for various numbers of non-recombinant and recombinant offspring in each family can be read off directly from the table. When the parents' phase is not known (as in two generation families) the z_1 score and its correction (e_1) have to be determined. The z_1 score is determined in the following manner. The offspring are divided up according to whether or not they possess the main character and/or the test character. In the example on p. 64 this would have been necessary if there had been no information on individuals in generation I. Thus:

Main character (G) + test character (T)　　 = 2 ⎫
(myotonic dystrophy + secretor)　　　　　　　　　 ⎬ 5
Not main character (g) + not test character (t) = 3 ⎭
(healthy + non-secretor)
Main character (G) + not test character (t)　 = 0 ⎫
(myotonic dystrophy + non-secretor)　　　　　　　 ⎬ 1
Not main character (g) + test character (T)　 = 1 ⎭
(healthy + secretor)

Thus the z_1 score is indicated as $5:1$ (the larger number is conventionally written first) and is looked up in tables under the heading 'z_1 5:1'. The e_1 correction is necessary only when the test character genotype of a parent can only be derived from an offspring involved in the count for z_1. It is equal to the number of individuals with or without the main character. In the above example this would be 4:2 (the larger number is again written first). The z_1 and e_1 scores, indicated as 'z_1 5:1' and 'e_1 4:2', are then obtained from Appendix 6 and would be added to the lod scores from other families.

The anti log of the sum of the lod scores for individual families for various values of θ gives the relative probability of linkage for each value of θ.

In extensive pedigrees of more than three generations the same logical approach is followed, the z_1 and e_1 scores are calculated and from these the lod scores are obtained.

The work involved however can be extremely tedious and time consuming and there is plenty of room for mistakes in logic particularly in extensive pedigrees. Fortunately computer programmes are now available for such computations (e.g. Freidhoff and Chase, 1975).

Prior probabilities of linkage

So far, we have considered that all values of the recombination fraction are equally likely. This is an oversimplification and Renwick (1969, 1971) has emphasized the need to take into account the initial or 'prior' probabilities of different values of θ.

Since chromosomes vary in length the probability that a given gene is located on a specific chromosome is proportional to the length of the chromosome. By considering the relative lengths of all 22 autosomes it has been calculated that the prior odds of linkage for any two genes, i.e. that two genes are located on the same autosome, is 1:17·5 (Renwick, 1969). Other prior odds to be considered include the differential rate of recombination in males and females (p. 70), known chromosomal location of one of the loci being studied and so on. To obtain the final odds for linkage the prior odds for each value of θ are taken into account. The calculation of prior probabilities is rather complicated and the reader is referred to the original papers by Renwick (1969, 1971). Fortunately, in practice, the inclusion of prior probabilities is not necessary if only a rough estimate of the recombination fraction is required and since human pedigree data are usually meagre, this is often all that is possible anyway.

Probability of linkage

The average height (H) of the relative probability curve indicates the odds on linkage, which for autosomal linkage are approximately equal to H:20. The average height of the relative probability curve is equal to the sum of the antilogs of the lod scores for $\theta = 0.05$,

0·10, 0·15 ··· 0·45 (Appendix 6) divided by 9. Thus if H is 100 then the odds on linkage would be 100 : 20 or 5 : 1.

Probability limits

The 0·95 *probability* limits (they are not really *confidence* limits in the true sense of the term) of the maximum likelihood estimate of the recombination fraction may be determined approximately by simply subtracting 2·5 per cent of the total area under the relative probability curve from each end of the curve. The total area of the curve may be determined by planimetry or simply by counting the number of one centimetre squares covered by the curve (see Fig. 6.7).

Recombination fraction and map distance

The relative distance between different loci on any particular chromosome is related to the frequency with which crossing-over occurs between them: one per cent crossing-over (i.e. $\theta = 0·01$) being equal to one map unit or centimorgan. The relationship between the recombination fraction and actual map distance however, is not linear. The farther apart the loci, the greater the discrepancy since double cross-overs will occur and be scored as non-recombinants. Several formulae have been derived which permit recombination fractions (for either autosomal or X-linkage) to be converted into map units. The formula of Kosambi (1944) is convenient

$$D = 25 \log_e \left(\frac{1 + 2\theta}{1 - 2\theta} \right)$$

where D = map distance in centimorgans
θ = recombination fraction.

If natural logarithms ($\log_e$) are not available then since $\log_e = 2·3026 \log_{10}$, therefore

$$D = 57·57 \log_{10} \left(\frac{1 + 2\theta}{1 - 2\theta} \right)$$

Because of the limitations to the amount of human data that are usually available, it is unlikely that linkage will be detectable if θ is much greater than 0·25.

Since the relationship between map distance and θ is essentially linear up to $\theta = 0·25$, from a practical point of view, recombination frequencies can be converted directly into map distances with little loss of precision.

For reasons which are not clear recombination is often greater in females than in males. Therefore in studying genetic linkage, if possible, families should be divided into those in which the mother is the doubly heterozygous parent and those in which the father is the doubly heterozygous parent and the recombination frequencies determined for males and females separately.

X-Linkage

Since no Mendelizing genes have yet been allocated to the Y chromosome, sex-linkage is synonymous with X-linkage. In assessing the linkage relationships between a main locus and a test locus, the offspring of doubly heterozygous females are scored. It has to be remembered, however, that if no one else in the family is affected a mother can only be considered heterozygous at the main locus (disease locus) if she has had at least two affected sons. If there is only one affected son this could be the result of a new mutation

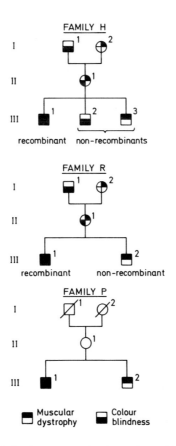

Fig. 6.6 Families in which Duchenne muscular dystrophy and deutan colour blindness are segregating. (From Emery, 1966.)

in which case the mother would not be a carrier. Of course if in a particular disorder there is a reliable test for the heterozygous state then even if the mother has only one affected son her genotype at the main locus can be firmly established as either GG or Gg.

Consider three families in which Duchenne muscular dystrophy (main character) and deutan colour blindness (test character) were segregating (Emery, 1966). In family H (Fig. 6.6) since the maternal grandfather was colour blind and his wife a carrier of Duchenne muscular dystrophy (she also had other male relatives with this disease) then these two loci must be in repulsion in their daughter II_1. Therefore III_1 must be a recombinant and III_2 and III_3 must be non-recombinants. Similarly in family R the mother (II_1) is doubly heterozygous and the colour blind and muscular dystrophy loci are in repulsion and therefore III_1 must be a recombinant and III_2 must be a non-recombinant.

In family P the grandfather (I_1) was dead. It was not known whether he was colour blind and therefore the linkage phase in the mother (II_1) is not known. In this case lod scores can be determined in the usual way. To determine the z_1 score (see p. 68):

$$\left. \begin{array}{ll} \textit{Main character (g)} + \text{test character }(t) & = 1 \\ \quad \text{(muscular dystrophy} + \text{colour blindness)} & \\ \text{Not main character }(G) + \text{not test character }(T) = 0 \\ \quad \text{(healthy} + \text{normal colour vision)} \end{array} \right\} 1$$

$$\left. \begin{array}{ll} \text{Main character }(g) + \text{not test character }(T) & = 1 \\ \quad \text{(muscular dystrophy} + \text{normal colour vision)} & \\ \text{Not main character }(G) + \text{test character }(t) & = 0 \\ \quad \text{(healthy} + \text{colour blindness)} \end{array} \right\} 1$$

Therefore the z_1 score is indicated as $1:1$. The number of individuals with the main character (muscular dystrophy, g) is 2, therefore the e_1 correction is indicated as $2:0$. For the appropriate number of scored children the lod scores for each of these three families in which Duchenne muscular dystrophy and deutan colour blindness are segregating can be determined (Appendix 6) and then added to each other. The results clearly indicate (Emery, Smith and Sanger, 1969) that the loci for Duchenne muscular dystrophy and deutan colour blindness are only loosely linked (Table 6.2).

In studying X-linkage there is obviously a selection of such 'informative' families which introduces a bias into the calculations which may alter the lod scores slightly. Edwards (1971) has studied this problem in detail and has provided a table of modified lod scores which takes into account different modes of ascertainment. For precision, ideally one should perhaps use Edwards' Tables. They are complicated however and most will find that for all practical purposes the lod scores in Appendix 6 are quite adequate and in fact give very similar results.

Table 6.2 Duchenne-type muscular dystrophy and deutan colour blindness: lod scores and antilogs (relative probabilities).

	Recombination fraction (θ)								
	0·05	0·10	0·15	0·20	0·25	0·30	0·35	0·40	0·45
Family H 2 non-rec.: 1 rec.	−0·442	−0·188	−0·062	0·010	0·051	0·070	0·073	0·061	0·037
Family R 1 non-rec.: 1 rec.	−0·721	−0·444	−0·292	−0·194	−0·125	−0·076	−0·041	−0·018	−0·004
Family P z_1 1:1; e_1 2:0	−0·584	−0·340	−0·215	−0·138	−0·087	−0·052	−0·028	−0·012	−0·003
Sum of lod scores	−1·747	−0·972	−0·569	−0·322	−0·161	−0·058	0·004	0·031	0·030
Antilog = relative probability	0·018	0·106	0·269	0·476	0·690	0·875	1·009	1·074	1·072

Table 6.3 Becker-type muscular dystrophy and deutan colour blindness: lod scores and antilogs (relative probabilities).

	Recombination fraction (θ)								
	0·05	0·10	0·15	0·20	0·25	0·30	0·35	0·40	0·45
Family E lod score	−2·94	−1·00	−0·08	0·41	0·64	0·69	0·62	0·45	0·23
Family M lod score	0·39	0·83	0·90	0·80	0·61	0·37	0·14	−0·01	−0·06
Sum of lod scores	−2·55	−0·17	0·82	1·21	1·25	1·06	0·76	0·44	0·17
Antilog = relative probability	0·003	0·676	6·61	16·22	17·78	11·48	5·75	2·75	1·48

In a study of two large families in which deutan colour blindness and X-linked Becker muscular dystrophy are segregating the lod scores obtained (Skinner, Smith and Emery, 1974) are given in Table 6.3 and the relative probabilities for various values of θ plotted in Figure 6.7. The maximum likelihood estimate of θ is 0·23. Further, the area under the curve is roughly 125 cm^2, one-fortieth (2·5 per cent) of which is 3·1 cm^2. Subtracting this from either end of the relative probability curve we obtain 0·95 probability limits for θ of approximately 0·13 to 0·43 (Fig. 6.7). Therefore since the colour blind locus is about 23 map

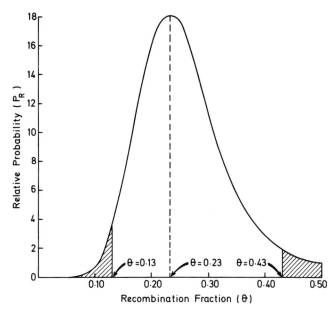

Fig. 6.7 Relative probabilities of linkage for various values of the recombination fraction for Becker muscular dystrophy and deutan colour blindness, and the 0·95 probability limits.

units from the locus for Becker muscular dystrophy but much further from the locus for Duchenne muscular dystrophy these results indicate that these two forms of X-linked muscular dystrophy are not allelic. Recently the locus for glucose-6-phosphate dehydrogenase (G6PD) has also been shown to be only loosely linked to the locus for Duchenne muscular dystrophy but is within measurable distance of the locus for Becker muscular dystrophy (Zatz et al., 1974). Since the loci for colour blindness and G6PD are known to be closely linked, this provides further evidence of the linkage relationships between these two forms of X-linked muscular dystrophy and colour blindness.

Note that by linkage studies it is possible to disprove allelism but because of their relative crudity in man, linkage studies can never be used to prove allelism.

Finally it should be appreciated that if the results of pedigree analysis suggest that two loci may be within measurable distance of each other, one will be more confident of the linkage relationship the greater the lod scores and the narrower the 0·95 probability limits.

7. Twin Studies, their Use and Limitations

Here we shall not be concerned so much with twinning as a biological phenomenon, which has been dealt with in detail by Bulmer (1970), but rather with the value of twin studies in genetic analysis. There are definitely two, and possibly three, types of twins. Firstly, there are dizygous (DZ), non-identical or fraternal twins derived from the independent release and subsequent fertilization of two separate ova. Such twins are genetically no more alike than sibs. Secondly, there are monozygous (MZ), or identical twins derived from the splitting of a single fertilized ovum at an early stage in development. They therefore have the same genotype and are of the same sex. A third type of twin resulting from the fertilization by two separate sperms of two division products of the *same* oocyte is theoretically possible but evidence of the existence in man is inconclusive. In man this form of fertilization usually results in a mosaic individual.

The frequency of MZ twinning is essentially the same throughout the world at about 1/285 births (3·5/1000), but whereas the frequency

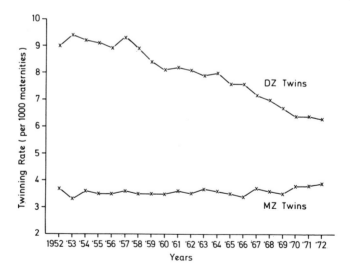

Fig. 7.1 Dizygotic (DZ) and monozygotic (MZ) twinning rates (per 1000 maternities) for England, Scotland and Wales.

of DZ twins in Western Europeans is about 6–9/1000 it is about twice this in Negroes and less than half this in Orientals. Also MZ twinning is little influenced by maternal age, parity or hereditary factors but the frequency of DZ twins increases significantly with parity, increases with maternal age reaching a maximum at 35 to 40 years (Bulmer, 1959), and depends on the mother's (but not the father's) genotype. There has been a gradual decline in the frequency of DZ twins (but not MZ twins) in the United Kingdom over the last 20 years (Fig. 7.1). Possible explanations for secular changes in dizygotic twinning rates have been discussed by James (1972) who has suggested that the cause may be more environmental rather than biological.

Diagnosis of zygosity

The first priority in twin studies is to establish the zygosity. There are essentially three ways of doing this. The first is a statistical method (so-called Weinberg's method) which is used to estimate the numbers of different types of twins. The other two methods are used for diagnosing the zygosity in individual twin pairs: one depends on the fetal membranes and the other on similarities between the twins.

Weinberg's method (Weinberg, 1901)
Since all MZ twins are of like-sex but half of DZ twins will be of unlike sex, then the number of DZ twins can be estimated by doubling the number of unlike-sex twins, and the number of MZ twins is the difference between the numbers of like-sexed and unlike-sexed twins.

Thus the proportion of DZ twins is

$$\frac{2U}{N}$$

where U = number of unlike-sexed twins
N = total number of maternities

and the proportion of MZ twins is

$$\frac{L - U}{N}$$

where L = number of like-sexed twins.

Therefore per 1000 maternities the DZ twinning rate is

$$\frac{2U}{N} \times 1000$$

and the MZ twinning rate

$$\frac{L - U}{N} \times 1000$$

Thus in 1973 in Scotland there were 74 500 maternities of which 747 resulted in twin births: 516 of like sex and 231 of unlike sex. Therefore the frequency of DZ twins is

$$\frac{2 \times 231}{74\ 500} \times 1000$$

$$= 6{\cdot}2 \text{ per 1000 maternities}$$

and the frequency of MZ twins is

$$\frac{516 - 231}{74\ 500} \times 1000$$

$$= 3{\cdot}8 \text{ per 1000 maternities.}$$

The frequency of multiple births very roughly follows Hellin's law. That is if the frequency of twins is t, the frequency of triplets is t^2, the frequency of quadruplets t^3, etc. However because multiple births may result from treatment with recently introduced 'fertility drugs' this simple relationship may now no longer hold.

Fetal membranes

Examination of the fetal membranes is the time-honoured method of diagnosing zygosity at birth. There are a number of possibilities which are summarized diagrammatically in Figure 7.2. In all cases where there is a single chorion (monochorionic) the twins are unequivocally MZ since this occurs in about 70 per cent of MZ twins but never in DZ twins. In other situations the diagnosis of zygosity is not clear cut and though dichorionic twins are more likely to be DZ, an individual dichorionic twin pair of like-sex cannot be unequivocally diagnosed by fetal membranes alone. For this reason and because information on fetal membranes may not always be available the so-called similarity method of diagnosing zygosity is often resorted to.

Similarity method

The object of this method is to compare, in the twin pair under study, traits in which MZ twins would be expected to resemble each other more closely than DZ twins. By such studies it is possible to estimate the relative probability of monozygosity to dizygosity. If a pair of twins differs in one simply inherited trait, such as sex, eye colour, or blood group, then the twins must be dizygotic. On the other hand, apart from skin grafting, a pair of twins can never be proved with certainty to be monozygotic, though with a large number of traits the probability that a twin pair is monozygotic may become almost unity. It should be remembered, however, that very rarely MZ twins may have a different phenotype or chromosome constitution as a result of post-zygotic aberrations (Nielsen, 1967; Benirschke and Kim, 1973).

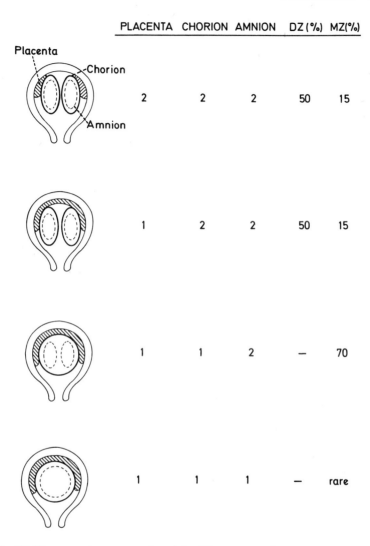

PLACENTA	CHORION	AMNION	DZ (%)	MZ(%)
2	2	2	50	15
1	2	2	50	15
1	1	2	—	70
1	1	1	—	rare

Fig. 7.2 Diagrammatic representation of the different types of placentation and their frequencies in DZ and MZ twins.

Techniques used in this method include blood group typing, determination of certain polymorphic phenotypes demonstrable in serum, erythrocytes and/or leucocytes, PTC tasting, secretor status and dermatoglyphics. The determination of zygosity using this method is much simpler when the parental phenotypes are known. The following example will illustrate the method of calculation. The findings in the father and mother of twin boys J and A were as follows:

	Father	Mother	J	A
Blood groups				
	O	A_1B	A_1	A_1
	R_1r	R_1R_1	R_1R_1	R_1R_1
	$MsNs$	$MsNs$	$MsNs$	$MsNs$
	P-pos	P-pos	P-pos	P-pos
	$Lu(a-)$	$Lu(a-)$	$Lu(a-)$	$Lu(a-)$
	$Kell$-neg	$Kell$-neg	$Kell$-neg	$Kell$-neg
	$Fy(a+)$	$Fy(a+)$	$Fy(a+)$	$Fy(a+)$
Secretor status	secretor	secretor	secretor	secretor
Haptoglobin type	1–1	2–1	2–1	2–1
Dermatoglyphics				
Total ridge count	—	—	161	165
Sum of atd angles	—	—	86°	88°

Clearly the only informative data are the ABO and Rhesus blood groups, haptoglobin types and dermatoglyphic findings. Since approximately 70 per cent of all twins are DZ, the *prior* probability that twins are DZ is 0·70 and the probability of their being MZ is 0·30. In the above example, the *conditional* (see p. 89) probabilities of the second twin having the same sex, ABO and Rh blood groups and haptoglobin type as the first twin if the twins are DZ is 0·50 in each case. From tables of dermatoglyphic findings in various types of twins (Smith and Penrose, 1955; Smith, Penrose and Smith, 1961), a difference in total ridge count of only four occurs in about 4 per cent of like-sexed DZ twins and 27 per cent of MZ twins, and a difference in atd angles of only 2° occurs in about 9 per cent of DZ twins and in 18 per cent of MZ twins.

The prior, and each of the individual conditional probabilities are multiplied together to give a *joint* probability of either dizygosity (JP_{DZ}) or monozygosity (JP_{MZ}). The probability of dizygosity is then

$$= \frac{JP_{DZ}}{JP_{DZ} + JP_{MZ}}$$

and the probability of monozygosity

$$= \frac{JP_{MZ}}{JP_{DZ} + JP_{MZ}}$$

or one minus the probability of dizygosity. In the above example the calculations are as follows:

Character	P_{DZ}	P_{MZ}
Prior probabilities	0·70	0·30
Conditional probabilities		
Sex	0·50	1·00
Blood groups		
ABO	0·50	1·00
Rh	0·50	1·00
Haptoglobin type	0·50	1·00
Dermatoglyphics		
diff. in TRC (4)	0·04	0·27
diff. in atd angles (2°)	0·09	0·18
Joint probability	0·0001575	0·01458

The probability of dizygosity is therefore

$$\frac{0\cdot0001575}{0\cdot0147375}$$

$$= 0\cdot0107$$

and the probability of monozygosity is

$$1 - 0\cdot0107$$

$$= 0\cdot9893.$$

In this case there is a 99 per cent probability that the twins are monozygous. It should be noted that with continuously variable traits such as dermatoglyphics, stature or cephalic index, a diagnosis of zygosity can never be made with certainty.

Now if we had had no information on the parents of these two twins then the probabilities of obtaining the various observed traits in the twins would have to have been based on gene frequencies in the general population. The calculations are very tedious but fortunately tables of relative probabilities of dizygosity are available (Smith and Penrose, 1955; Smith et al., 1961), for blood groups and some other traits based on their population frequencies in the United Kingdom. With such information the method of calculation is as follows. If p_0D, p_1D, p_2D, etc. are the relative probabilities of dizygosity for each trait under consideration, then the overall relative probability of dizygosity (pD) based on this information is

$$= p_0D \times p_1D \times p_2D \times \ldots$$

and the total probability of the twins being dizygous is

$$= pD/(1 + pD)$$

and the probability of the twins being monozygous is

$$= 1 - [pD/(1 + pD)]$$

Thus in the above example:

Character	Relative probability of dizygosity
Prior prob.	2·3333 (i.e. 0·7/0·3)
Like-sex	0·5000
Blood groups	
ABO (A_1)	0·6470
Rh (R_1R_1)	0·5021
MNS (MNss)	0·4733
P ($P+$)	0·8489
Lu ($A-$)	0·9614
K ($K-$)	0·9485
Fy ($a+$)	0·8036
Secretor status	
secretor	0·8681
Dermatoglyphics	
Total ridge count	0·23
atd angles	0·50
Relative probability of dizygosity (pD)	0·01114

The probability of dizygosity is therefore

$$\frac{0·01114}{1·01114}$$

$$= 0·0110$$

and the probability of monozygosity is

$$1 - 0·0110$$

$$= 0·9890$$

Gaines and Elston (1969) have produced a series of curves (Fig. 7.3) from which it is possible to read off directly the relative probability of dizygosity for any gene frequency (q) and which are therefore applicable to any simply inherited trait in any population in which the gene frequency is known. Curve A is used when the twins are homozygous as when one of the two alleles is dominant and the twins have the recessive phenotype, or if the two alleles are codominant and the twins have the phenotype of either of the two homozygous genotypes. Here 'q' is the frequency of the *common* allele. Curve B is used when the twins are heterozygous as when the two alleles are codominant and the twins have the heterozygous phenotype. Here 'q'

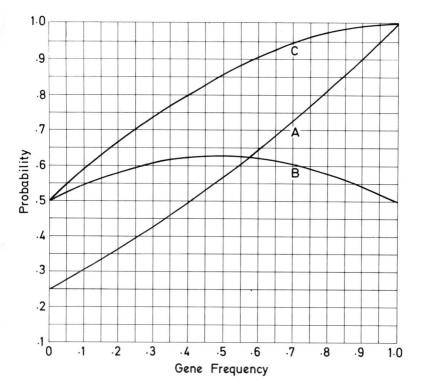

Fig. 7.3 Relative probability of dizygosity as a function of gene frequency (q). For details see text. (From Gaines and Elston, 1969.)

is the frequency of *either* allele. Curve C is used when the twins could be either homozygous or heterzygous as when one allele is dominant and the twins exhibit the phenotype associated with the dominant allele. Here 'q' is the frequency of the *dominant* allele. Thus in the above example, the $P+$ phenotype represents the homozygote PP or the heterozygote Pp, the gene frequency of P being about 0·50 in Western Europe. Therefore from curve C the relative probability of dizygosity is about 0·86.

The use of twins in genetic analysis

The main value of twin studies in genetic analysis is that they can give an idea of the role of genetic factors in aetiology. From this point of view the most commonly employed techniques are the study of *concordance rates* (for discontinuous characters such as disease states) and *variances* and *correlations* (for continuous characters such as serum lipoproteins).

Concordance rates

If both twins of a pair are affected they are said to be concordant, while if only one twin is affected they are said to be discordant. Concordance rates can be defined in a number of ways (Allen, Harvald and Shields, 1967). Firstly there is the *pairwise concordance* rate (C_w) which may be defined as the proportion of affected twin pairs in which *both* members are affected. The pairwise concordance rate is usually given by

$$\frac{C}{C + D}$$

where $C = total$ number of concordant pairs
$\quad\quad\quad D =$ number of discordant pairs.

Thus in one recent study of schizophrenia in twins (Gottesman and Shields, 1972) there were 11 concordant and 11 discordant pairs of MZ twins and 3 concordant and 30 discordant pairs of DZ twins. Therefore

$$C_wMZ = 11/22 = 50 \text{ per cent}$$

$$C_wDZ = \;\;3/33 = \;\;9 \text{ per cent.}$$

Concordance may also be expressed as the *proband concordance* rate (C_p) which may be defined as the proportion of affected individuals among the co-twins of previously ascertained index cases. When both twins are affected and have been independently ascertained, the twin pair is in effect counted twice. The proband concordance rate is given by

$$\frac{C + C'}{C + D + C'}$$

where $C' =$ number of concordant pairs ascertained *independently* through *both* affected twins.

Thus in the above example of the 11 concordant pairs of MZ twins, both of the affected co-twins were ascertained independently in four pairs, and of the three concordant pairs of DZ twins in one pair both twins had been ascertained independently.
Therefore

$$C_pMZ = \frac{11 + 4}{11 + 11 + 4} = 58 \text{ per cent}$$

$$C_pDZ = \frac{3 + 1}{3 + 30 + 1} = 12 \text{ per cent}$$

It should be noted that if an attempt is made to ascertain *all* affected twins in the population then $C = C'$ and therefore

$$C_p = \frac{2C'}{2C' + D}$$

Thus by attempting complete ascertainment of all affected twins, this gets around the problem of deciding whether or not a pair of concordant twins have been independently ascertained. It can also be shown (Smith, 1972a) that if *all* twins with the trait in question have been ascertained then

$$C_w = C_p/(2 - C_p)$$

and

$$C_p = 2C_w/(1 + C_w)$$

so the two concordance rates can be derived one from the other. If the condition under consideration is comparatively uncommon and/or ascertainment is low, no pair of twins is likely to be doubly ascertained ($C' = 0$) and therefore the two concordance rates are equivalent.

On balance the proband concordance rate is to be preferred to the pairwise concordance rate for reasons which are discussed in detail by Allen *et al.* (1967). Unfortunately in many twin studies in the past the mode of ascertainment was either not recorded or not taken into account.

. The interpretation put on concordance rates is that for a disorder in which genetic factors are important in aetiology, the concordance rate for MZ twins reared apart will be about the same as for MZ twins reared together, and the concordance rate for MZ twins will be greater than for DZ twins. As was discussed earlier it is possible to estimate from concordance rates the correlation in liability between twins and form this it is possible to derive the heritability (p. 60). Again it must be emphasized that if the frequency of a disorder is low (i.e. 0·1 per cent or less), the concordance rate in MZ twins will also be low unless the heritability is very high (Smith, 1970).

Variances and correlations

An idea of the degree of genetic influence on a continuously variable trait may be gauged from the intra (within)-pair and inter (between)-pair variances (Osborne and De George, 1959) and the intraclass correlation.

The intrapair variance

$$= \frac{\Sigma (A - B)^2}{2N}$$

which has N degrees of freedom.

The interpair variance

$$= \frac{1}{N-1}\left[\frac{\Sigma(A+B)^2}{2} - \frac{[\Sigma(A+B)]^2}{2N}\right]$$

which has $N - 1$ degrees of freedom, where

N = number of twin pairs
A and B = values for the members of each twin pair.

Variances may be compared by dividing the larger by the smaller the ratio being referred to as 'F', the statistical significance of which can be determined from reference to standard tables of 'F' values (Fisher and Yates, 1963).

The method of calculation is illustrated from some data on serum cholesterol levels in twins (Osborne et al., 1959).

Since a trait such as serum cholesterol level may well be affected by age, sex and environmental factors and for the sake of simplicity in merely wishing to demonstrate the method of calculation, only the authors' data on adult male twins reared together will be considered. Their figures have been rounded-off to one decimal place. For MZ twins the intrapair variance was 279·5 ($N = 14$) and the interpair variance was 2780·5 ($N = 18$). For DZ twins the intrapair variance was 694·3 ($N = 6$) and the interpair variance was 1519·1 ($N = 6$). Thus comparing the *interpair* variances of MZ and DZ twins (MZ/DZ):

$$F = \frac{2780 \cdot 5}{1519 \cdot 1}$$

$$= 1 \cdot 83$$

Whereas comparing the *intrapair* variances of MZ and DZ twins (DZ/MZ):

$$F = \frac{694 \cdot 3}{279 \cdot 5}$$

$$= 2 \cdot 48$$

Neither of these 'F' values is statistically significant but since the intrapair variance for DZ twins is more than twice that for MZ twins, this suggests that hereditary factors play a role in the control of normal serum cholesterol levels.

However though intrapair and interpair variances can give an idea of the role of genetic factors in aetiology, they are not in themselves a measure of the degree of genetic determination.

Another approach to the problem is to measure the correlation between pairs of twins, but it is not possible to calculate the usual correlation coefficient because there is no way of deciding which measurement on a pair of twins is X and which is Y. For this reason a different type of correlation coefficient is determined. This is referred to as the *intraclass correlation coefficient* (r) which treats the pairs of measurements symmetrically. It is equal to

$$\frac{\text{interpair variance} - \text{intrapair variance}}{\text{interpair variance} + \text{intrapair variance}}$$

From the intraclass correlation coefficient it is then possible to calculate the heritability (p. 53) since

$$h^2 = r/R$$

where R = coefficient of relationship

Therefore for MZ twins

$$h^2 = r$$

and for DZ twins

$$h^2 = 2r$$

In the above example the intraclass correlation for male MZ twins reared together

$$= \frac{2780 \cdot 5 - 279 \cdot 5}{2780 \cdot 5 + 279 \cdot 5}$$

$$= 0 \cdot 82$$

therefore $h^2 = 82$ per cent

The intraclass correlation for male DZ twins reared together

$$= \frac{1519 \cdot 1 - 694 \cdot 3}{1519 \cdot 1 + 694 \cdot 3}$$

$$= 0 \cdot 37$$

therefore $h^2 = 74$ per cent.

Problems and limitations of twin studies

Twin studies have been helpful in fostering a great deal of research. The results of such studies have emphasized the role of genetic factors in aetiology in a variety of conditions. However there are limitations, both statistical and biological, to the twin method. The statistical problems are those of ascertainment and the interpretation to be placed upon such parameters as intrapair and interpair variances. Edwards (1968) has argued that since all diseases have some genetic predisposition the estimation of such parameters may be a costly way of confirming expectations without providing any useful measure of the intensity of this predisposition. However, recent studies have shown that concordance rates and intraclass correlations can be used to estimate the heritability which is meaningful in terms of measuring the degree of genetic determination.

In the literature much use has been made of an index attributed to Holzinger (1929) as estimating the degree of genetic determination from twin data. This index, often referred to as 'H', has been variously expressed in terms of concordance rates:

$$(C_{MZ} - C_{DZ})/(1 - C_{DZ})$$

in terms of intraclass correlations:

$$(r_{MZ} - r_{DZ})/(1 - r_{DZ})$$

and in terms of intrapair variances:

$$(V_{DZ} - V_{MZ})/V_{DZ}$$

However, this 'H' index is an arbitrary index and has no specific genetic interpretation (Cavalli-Sforza and Bodmer, 1971). It is not an estimate of heritability and should therefore not be used for this purpose. For these reasons it has been recommended that the use of the 'H' index should be discontinued (Smith, 1974).

The biological limitations to the twin method are more complex and difficult to cater for. They include prenatal factors such as position *in utero,* manner of delivery, and the possibility of shared placental circulation, as well as postnatal factors and perhaps here the main problem is the tendency for twins to share the same environment. It is for this latter reason that comparisons between MZ twins reared together and reared apart can be helpful.

It has been suggested by some that the twin method has not vindicated the time spent on the collection of such data. This may have been true to some extent. Certainly considerable care is needed in the collection, analysis and interpretation of twin data.

8. Estimation of Recurrence Risks for Genetic Counselling

Recurrence risks are based upon either Mendelian principles, in the case of unifactorial disorders, or empiric observations on the frequency of a particular disorder among relatives of affected individuals in the case of multifactorial disorders. The estimation of recurrence risks in both these situations has been discussed in detail by Murphy and Chase (1975). Here we shall only be concerned with the principles of such calculations.

Unifactorial disorders

When considering the probability of an individual having a particular genotype (preclinical case or a heterozygous carrier) it is customary to base such calculations on 'anterior' information only. That is the *prior* probability based on knowledge of the individual's antecedents and sibs. But this ignores 'posterior' information based on the individual's phenotype (clinical findings and test results) and that of any of the individual's offspring. From such posterior information it is possible to calculate so-called *conditional* probabilities. The product of the prior and conditional probabilities is the *joint* probability. The final *posterior* probability of an individual having a particular genotype is the joint probability of getting the observed information given the genotype in question, divided by the sum of this probability and the joint probability of getting the observed information if the individual is normal.

The expression of posterior probabilities in terms of prior and conditional probabilities in this way is known as Bayes' theorem or Bayes' law (Bayes, 1763).

In general terms, if the prior probability of an event A occurring is denoted as $P(A)$, and of A not occurring as $P(\text{not } A)$, and if the conditional probability of event O if A occurs (i.e. probability of O given A) is $P(O \mid A)$, and if the conditional probability of event O if A does not occur is $P(O \mid \text{not } A)$, then the probability of A given O

$$P(A \mid O) = \frac{P(A)P(O \mid A)}{P(A)P(O \mid A) + P(\text{not } A)P(O \mid \text{not } A)}$$

This is illustrated in the case of an apparently healthy man aged 50 whose father died of Huntington's chorea and who wishes to know if his own son may one day become affected. This disorder is inherited as an autosomal dominant trait, the first signs of which usually appear sometime between the ages of 25 and 55. The prior probability of having inherited the disorder from his father is 1/2. Since approximately 80 per cent of cases of Huntington's chorea develop symptoms before the age of 50, the chance (conditional probability) that he would not have manifested the disease by this age even if he had inherited the gene is about 20 per cent (1/5). Therefore the joint probability of having inherited the disease and being clinically unaffected at age 50 is 1/10. The prior probability of not having inherited the disease is 1/2 and of course the conditional probability of being normal if he has *not* inherited the gene is 1, and therefore the joint probability is 1/2. The posterior probability of having inherited the disease given that he is apparently unaffected at age 50 is therefore 1/6:

Probability	Inherited the disorder	Not inherited the disorder
Prior	1/2	1/2
Conditional	1/5	1
Joint	1/10	1/2
Posterior	$\dfrac{1/10}{1/10 + 1/2} \simeq 1/6$	

The prior probability that his son will have inherited the gene is therefore 1 in 12 or 8·5 per cent. Of course as each year goes by and the father and son remain healthy so their risks of having inherited the gene decrease. The probabilities that an apparently healthy individual and his or her offspring may have inherited Huntington's chorea, polyposis coli or myotonic dystrophy have been calculated in this way from data (based on clinical findings) in the literature and from personal studies and the results expressed graphically in Figures 8.1, 8.2 and 8.3, respectively.

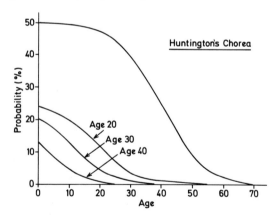

Fig. 8.1 Probability that an apparently healthy parent and offspring (born when the still unaffected parent was aged 20, 30 and 40 years) may have inherited Huntington's chorea from an affected grandparent.

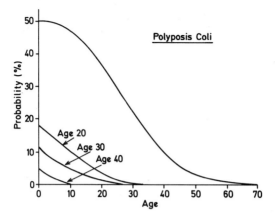

Fig. 8.2 Probability that an apparently healthy parent and offspring (born when the still unaffected parent was aged 20, 30 and 40 years) may have inherited polyposis coli from an affected grandparent.

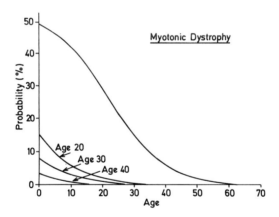

Fig. 8.3 Probability that an apparently healthy parent and offspring (born when the still unaffected parent was aged 20, 30 and 40 years) may have inherited myotonic dystrophy from an affected grandparent.

This Bayesian approach to probability calculations and the estimation of genetic risks has been eloquently discussed by Murphy and Mutalik (1969). The method is particularly valuable in the case of X-linked recessive disorders where the problem is to determine the probability of a particular woman being a carrier. The detection of symptomless female carriers is an important problem in genetic counselling. During recent years a number of tests have been devised by means of which it is possible to detect carriers of X-linked recessive disorders. Unfortunately, in some of these tests there is overlap in the results obtained in known carriers and normal women in which case a suspected carrier with a normal test result presents a particularly difficult problem and it is in this regard that Bayesian methods can be particularly helpful.

Of course if an appropriate test indicates that a woman is a definite carrier, then genetic counselling can be based on first principles and this more elaborate approach is not necessary.

In a lethal X-linked disorder, such as Duchenne muscular dystrophy, the prior probability of any woman being a carrier is 4μ (p. 30). If a suspected carrier has two sons one of whom is affected, the conditional probability of this, assuming she is a carrier, is $1/4$, and if she is not a carrier is μ (the affected son being a new mutation). Now in the case of Duchenne muscular dystrophy approximately two-thirds of known carriers have a serum level of creatine kinase which exceeds the normal 95 percentile (Emery, 1965). If a suspected carrier's serum level of creatine kinase is therefore less than the normal 95 percentile then the conditional probability of this if she is a carrier is $1/3$ and if she is not a carrier is $19/20$. Thus:

Probability	Carrier	Not a carrier
Prior	4μ	$1-4\mu \simeq 1$
Conditional 　　genetic 　　biochemical	$(1/2)^2$ $1/3$	μ $19/20$
Joint	$\mu/3$	$\mu 19/20$

Posterior	$\dfrac{\mu/3}{\mu/3 + \mu 19/20} = 0 \cdot 26$

A general formula for calculating the probability of a woman being a carrier of a lethal X-linked disorder, which affects either a brother or a son, has been derived (Emery and Morton, 1968). If h_c and h_m, based on the results of biochemical and other tests, refer respectively to the relative probabilities of normal homozygosity to heterozygosity in the suspected carrier and her mother, so that if there is no such information $h = 1$,

and if　q = number of normal brothers
and　　r = number of normal sons
and if　$s = 1$ where a son is affected and 0 if a brother is affected
and　　$t = 0$ where a son is affected and 1 if a brother is affected

then the probability (P) of her being a carrier of a *lethal* X-linked disorder:

$$P = \frac{1 + sa}{1 + sa + ab + tb}$$

where

$$a = h_m 2^q$$

and

$$b = h_c 2^r$$

If the frequency of carrier females is $H\mu$ (i.e. 4μ when the fitness of affected males is 0, as in Duchenne muscular dystrophy, or 18μ when the fitness of affected males is 0·7, as in haemophilia A (see p. 31)) then the probability of a woman being a carrier of any X-linked disorder:

$$P = \frac{1 + sa'}{1 + sa' + a'b + tb}$$

where

$$a' = a4/H$$

For example in the case of haemophilia A where $H = 18\mu$

$$a' = a\,4/18$$

$$= 0 \cdot 22a$$

therefore

$$P = \frac{1 + 0 \cdot 22sa}{1 + 0 \cdot 22sa + 0 \cdot 22ab + tb}$$

The relative probabilities of normal homozygosity to heterozygosity (h) can be estimated by simply classifying the data according to an arbitrary upper limit of normal as was done in the above example where for a serum level of creatine kinase *below* the normal 95 percentile

$$h = 0 \cdot 95/0 \cdot 33$$

$$= 2 \cdot 88$$

This is inefficient however, because not all the information is being used and it would seem better to estimate 'h' from the *actual* values of the particular character being measured. For example, by taking into account the suspected carriers actual serum level of creatine kinase and comparing this with values in normal women. This can be done by calculating the ratio of the proportion of normal women to the proportion of known carriers who have a particular serum level of creatine kinase as shown in Table 8.1.

To illustrate how the probability of a woman being a carrier is calculated, consider the case of a suspected carrier who has a *brother* with Duchenne muscular dystrophy $(s = 0; t = 1)$, two normal brothers $(q = 2)$ and one normal son $(r = 1)$. Her serum level of creatine kinase

Table 8.1 Relative probabilities of normal homozygosity to heterozygosity ('h') for various serum levels of creatine kinase expressed in International Units.

Serum creatine kinase (IU)	Controls		Carriers		h
	No.	% (Y_1)	No.	% (Y_2)	(Y_1/Y_2)
11–20	34	28·3	2	3·6	7·86
21–30	55	45·8	5	9·1	5·03
31–40	15	12·5	3	5·5	2·27
41–50	8	6·7	7	12·7	0·53
51–60	6	5·0	6	10·9	0·46
61–70	2	1·7	3	5·5	0·31
> 70	—	—	29	52·7	—
Total	120	100·0	55	100·0	—

is 25 IU ($h_c = 5·03$) and her mother's serum level of creatine kinase is 35 IU ($h_m = 2·27$). Therefore her probability of being a carrier is

$$= \frac{1 + s h_m 2^q}{1 + s h_m 2^q + h_m 2^q h_c 2^r + t h_c 2^r}$$

but $\qquad s = 0 \quad \text{and} \quad t = 1$

therefore $\qquad P = \dfrac{1}{1 + h_m 2^q h_c 2^r + h_c 2^r}$

$$= \frac{1}{1 + (2·27)(2)^2(5·03)(2) + (5·03)(2)}$$

$$= \frac{1}{102·4}$$

or approximately 1 per cent.

Thus, in order to give reliable genetic counselling to a suspected carrier of an X-linked disorder, such as Duchenne muscular dystrophy, who has only one affected male relative it is important to know how many normal sons and brothers she has. It is also very important to know not only her serum level of creatine kinase *but also her mother's*.

One further complication however requires consideration. In the Becker type of X-linked muscular dystrophy serum levels of creatine kinase decrease with age in carriers, which means that in this disorder in determining the probability of a woman being a carrier her age as well as her serum level of creatine kinase must be taken into account (Skinner *et al.*, 1975).

The method given above for calculating 'h' values and the general principles involved apply to any X-linked disorder where quantitative data on carriers are available. For example, factor VIII and factor VIII-like antigen in carriers of haemophilia A. Further, the results of different tests may be combined by multiplying together 'h' values from the different tests. For example, combining data from serum levels of creatine kinase and electromyography in the case of a suspected carrier of Duchenne muscular dystrophy. Thus a woman who has an affected *brother,* but no other brothers and no sons, and if two different tests have yielded values of h_1 and h_2, then the probability of her being a carrier is

$$\frac{1}{1 + 2h_1h_2}$$

If the problem had been that she had an affected *son,* but no brothers and no other children, then the probability would have been

$$\frac{1}{1 + (h_1h_2)/2}$$
$$= \frac{2}{2 + h_1h_2}$$

It should be noted however, that it is only legitimate to multiply h_1 and h_2 if the two tests are statistically independent, i.e. they are not positively correlated for controls or carriers.

In conclusion, the Bayesian method of calculating probabilities, based on estimating values of 'h', can provide little information if the data are limited and is unnecessary when the results of a particular test indicate a clear dichotomy between normal women and carriers. The method is most valuable in those X-linked disorders where there is overlap in test results in normal women and carriers. The particular method chosen for estimating 'h' will depend upon the amount of data available. As we have seen, values for 'h' can be estimated from an arbitrary classification into normal and abnormal if the data are limited, or from density functions if the data are extensive.

Multifactorial disorders

By determining the frequency of a particular disorder among relatives it is possible to predict recurrence risks, for example, to children born subsequent to an affected child in a family. Such information is also important in segregation analysis when unifactorial inheritance is suspected (see Chapter 4) or for calculating the heritability when multifactorial inheritance is suspected (p. 53).

Empiric risk figures for sibs may be determined by considering the proportion of affected individuals among *all* sibs as is usually done in segregation analysis. However this assumes that the risks to children born before the proband are no different from the risks to children born after the proband. This is true for unifactorial disorders but

Table 8.2 Empiric risks for some common disorders (in per cent) (*From* Emery, A. E. H., 1975).

Disorder	Incidence	Sex ratio M : F	Normal parents having a second affected child	Affected parent having an affected child	Affected parent having a second affected child
Anencephaly	0·20	1 : 2	2	—	—
Cleft palate only	0·04	2 : 3	2	7	15
Cleft lip ± cleft palate	0·10	3 : 2	4	4	10
Club foot	0·10	2 : 1	3	3	10
Cong. heart disease (all types)	0·50	—	1–4	1–4	—
Diabetes mellitus (early onset)	0·20	1 : 1	8	8	10
Dislocation of hip	0·10	1 : 6	4	4	10
Epilepsy ('idiopathic')	0·50	1 : 1	5	5	10
Hirschsprung's disease	0·02	4 : 1			
male index			2	—	—
female index			8	—	—
Manic-depressive psychoses	0·40	2 : 3	—	10–15	—
Mental retardation ('idiopathic')	0·30	1 : 1	3–5	—	—
Profound childhood deafness	0·10	1 : 1	10	6	—
Pyloric stenosis	0·30	5 : 1			
male index			2	4	13
female index			10	17	38
Schizophrenia	1–2	1 : 1	—	16	—
Scoliosis (idiopathic, adolescent)	0·22	1 : 6	7	5	—
Spina bifida	0·30	2 : 3	4	3	—

may not be true in other situations. For example, if there is the possibility that the recurrence of the disorder may be related to maternal age or birth order. This problem is illustrated in the case of endocardial fibroelastosis a disorder characterized by progressive cardiac failure beginning in early childhood and associated with gross cardiomegaly and characteristic cardiac histology, either at biopsy but usually at autopsy. The cause is not known, but various suggestions have been proposed including autoimmunity, viral infection, a recessive metabolic disorder or a multifactorial aetiology. In an extensive study of 119 families with this disorder, Chen and her colleagues (Chen, Thompson and Rose, 1971) found that whereas the frequency of the disorder in the general population is about 0·017 per cent, the frequency among *all* sibs was 3·8 per cent compared with a frequency of 17·7 per cent among sibs born *subsequent* to the index cases. The latter figure is clearly the appropriate one for genetic counselling when parents have already had an affected child. Therefore when determining empiric risks for genetic counselling purposes it is clearly important first of all to exclude the possibilities of a parental age or birth order effect on the recurrence in subsequent sibs. It would be ideal to base recurrence risks always on the frequency in subsequent sibs. However, in practice, this is often difficult because family limitation, subsequent to the birth of an affected child, may result in insufficient data being available.

Risk tables for genetic counselling in various family situations for cleft lip $+/-$ cleft palate, pyloric stenosis and CNS malformations are available (Bonaiti-Pellié and Smith, 1974). For some relatively common disorders empiric risks to sibs and to the children of affected individuals are given in Table 8.2. These are average figures but are usually adequate for genetic counselling purposes. In complex family situations there are computer programmes for risk calculations for unifactorial disorders, e.g. PEDIG (Heuch and Li, 1972; Conneally and Heuch, 1974) and multifactorial disorders, e.g. RISKMF (Smith, 1972b).

9. Disease Associations

One approach to demonstrating the role of genetic factors in the aetiology of a disorder is to determine if there is any association with an inherited marker trait such as a particular blood group or HLA type. If a disorder is found to be associated with a particular marker more frequently than would be expected by chance, this may suggest a causal relationship, that is the association may be due to multiple effects of the same gene. It should be remembered, however, that association can be due to other causes which include epistatic interaction (e.g. between the Lewis and secretor loci), selective interaction (e.g. between G6PD deficiency, thalassaemia and resistance to malaria in certain areas of the Mediterranean), population stratification (p. 104) and very close linkage resulting in 'linkage disequilibrium' that is certain alleles at adjacent loci are preferentially maintained in coupling (Bodmer *et al.*, 1969).

The first large-scale study of association was made by the late Professor Aird and his colleagues in 1953 (Aird, Bentall and Roberts, 1953). He had proposed that since cancer of the stomach and blood group O were both commoner in the North of England the two might be associated. In fact the association proved to be not with group O but with group A and the association was highly significant in all parts of the country. Since then, there have been many studies of disease associations either with blood groups (Roberts, 1957; Clarke, 1961; Vogel and Helmbold, 1972) or more recently with HLA types (McDevitt and Bodmer, 1974; Svejgaard *et al.*, 1975).

Statistical analysis

To determine the statistical significance of an association the method most widely used is that of Woolf (1955). This method has the advantage that it allows us to combine data from various centres, in which the marker trait may have different incidences, and it also allows us to test for heterogeneity between centres. The method involves essentially four steps.

1. The relative incidence
The patients and controls are divided into two groups depending on whether they have a particular marker (say α) or not (either β or not α). For example, those with blood group O as compared to those with blood group A, or those without group O (A, B and AB).

The relative incidence of the disease in persons with marker α compared to persons with marker β is obtained by cross-multiplication. Thus if

h = number of patients with marker α
H = number of controls with marker α
k = number of patients with marker β
K = number of controls with marker β

then we can draw up a table thus:

marker	patients	controls
α	h	H
β	k	K

and the relative incidence ('x') of the marker α in patients

$$= \frac{hK}{Hk}$$

For example in a large study in Liverpool there were 505 O's and 263 A's among patients with duodenal ulcer, and 7536 O's and 6013 A's in controls (Clarke, 1961). The relative incidence of duodenal ulcer in persons with group O compared to 1 in persons of group A is therefore

$$\frac{505 \times 6013}{7536 \times 263}$$

$$= 1\cdot53$$

To test the significance of this finding and in order to combine results from different centres it is necessary to calculate the *total* χ^2, *pooled* χ^2 and *heterogeneity* χ^2 (for the significance of which see Appendix 2, p. 132).

2. *Total* χ^2

If the relative incidence (x)

$$= \frac{hK}{Hk}$$

and if
$$y = \log_e x$$

and
$$w = \frac{1}{\dfrac{1}{h} + \dfrac{1}{k} + \dfrac{1}{H} + \dfrac{1}{K}}$$

then the significance of 'y' in individual studies is determined by calculating χ^2 for each study which is equal to wy^2 with one degree of freedom. χ^2 values for individual studies are then summed to give the *total* χ^2 ($= \Sigma wy^2$), the number of degrees of freedom of which is equal to the number of studies being combined.

3. Pooled χ^2

This tests the significance of the overall mean value of 'x' from unity and is equal to

$$\frac{(\Sigma wy)^2}{\Sigma w}$$

and has one degree of freedom.

4. Heterogeneity χ^2

This tests the departure of individual values of 'x' from the overall mean. It is obtained by subtracting the pooled χ^2 from the total χ^2:

$$\Sigma wy^2 - \frac{(\Sigma wy)^2}{\Sigma w}$$

The number of degrees of freedom is one less than the number of studies being combined.

In combining data from several studies the weighted estimated mean value of 'x' is the natural antilogarithm of $\Sigma wy/\Sigma w$ and its s.e. is the natural antilogarithm of $\sqrt{1/\Sigma w}$.

The method of calculation is illustrated with data from various centres in the U.K. on the association of peptic ulcer and blood group O (Woolf, 1955). The data and related calculations are summarized in Table 9.1. The results indicate that in all three centres there is a significant association between peptic ulcer and blood group O.

The pooled χ^2

$$= \frac{(\Sigma wy)^2}{\Sigma w}$$

$$= \frac{(189 \cdot 94)^2}{576 \cdot 0}$$

$$= 62 \cdot 63$$

and heterogeneity χ^2

$$= \Sigma wy^2 - \frac{(\Sigma wy)^2}{\Sigma w}$$

$$= 65 \cdot 62 - 62 \cdot 63$$

$$= 2 \cdot 99$$

With two degrees of freedom $0 \cdot 2 < P < 0 \cdot 3$. Therefore there is no apparent heterogeneity in the results of the three studies, which may therefore be combined.

Table 9.1 The association of peptic ulcer and blood group O relative to blood group A (Woolf, 1955)

| Centre | Peptic ulcer | | Controls | | $x = \dfrac{hK}{Hk}$ | $y = \log_e x$ | w^* | wy | $\chi^2 = wy^2$ | P |
	group O (h)	group A (k)	group O (H)	group A (K)						
London	911	579	4578	4219	1·4500	0·3716	304·9	113·30	42·11	<0·001
Manchester	361	246	4532	3775	1·2224	0·2008	136·6	27·43	5·50	<0·02
Newcastle	396	219	6598	5261	1·4418	0·3659	134·5	49·21	18·01	<0·001
						Sum	576·0	189·94	65·62	—

$$* w = \frac{1}{\dfrac{1}{h} + \dfrac{1}{k} + \dfrac{1}{H} + \dfrac{1}{K}}$$

Table 9.2 The association of ankylosing spondylitis with HLA antigen B 27. Data from London (Brewerton et al., 1973) and Los Angeles (Schlosstein et al., 1973)

| Centre | Ankylosing spondylitis | | Controls | | $x = \dfrac{hK}{Hk}$ | $y = \log_e x$ | w | wy | $\chi^2 = wy^2$ | P |
	B 27 (h)	not B 27 (k)	B 27 (H)	not B 27 (K)						
London	72	3	3	72	576·00	6·36	1·44	9·16	58·25	<0·001
Los Angeles	35	5	72	834	81·08	4·40	4·10	18·04	79·38	<0·001
						Sum	5·54	27·20	137·63	—

The weighted mean value of 'x' is the natural antilogarithm of

$$\frac{\Sigma wy}{\Sigma w}$$

$$= \frac{189\cdot94}{576\cdot0}$$

$$= 0\cdot33, \text{ the natural antilogarithm of}$$
which is $1\cdot39$.

Its s.e. is the natural antilogarithm of

$$\sqrt{1/\Sigma w}$$

$$= \sqrt{1/576\cdot0}$$

$$= 0\cdot0417$$

The 95 per cent confidence limits are therefore

$$0\cdot33 \pm (1\cdot96)(0\cdot0417)$$

$$= 0\cdot25 \text{ to } 0\cdot41$$

Taking natural antilogarithms the 95 per cent confidence limits are $1\cdot28$ to $1\cdot51$.

Another instructive example is afforded by data from Los Angeles (Schlosstein *et al.*, 1973) and London (Brewerton *et al.*, 1973) on the association between ankylosing spondylitis and the HLA antigen B 27 (Table 9.2). Clearly both studies reveal a highly significant association. Here the total χ^2 is $137\cdot63$, and the pooled χ^2 is $(27\cdot20)^2/5\cdot54$ or $133\cdot55$. The heterogeneity χ^2 is therefore

$$= 137\cdot63 - 133\cdot55$$

$$= 4\cdot08$$

With one degree of freedom this value of χ^2 is just significant ($0\cdot02 < P < 0\cdot05$). There is therefore a suggestion of heterogeneity in the data and it may not be entirely justified to combine the data from these two studies. However if one does, the weighted estimated mean value of the relative incidence is 135 (the natural antilogarithm of $27\cdot20/5\cdot54$ or $4\cdot91$). Therefore this association is very much greater than has been observed in the case of any of the blood group associations.

Analysis of sibships

Another approach to the problem of disease associations is Professor C. A. B. Smith's method of analysing sibships (*see* Clarke, 1959a, 1961). The principle of this method is to assess in each sibship in which the particular marker trait under consideration is segregating (in which some sibs have marker trait α and some β) the probability of the proband (the individual with the particular disorder under consideration) having marker trait α and then compare the total 'observed' results with the total 'expected'. Thus in a sibship of four in which two are of group O and two of group A, the 'expected' probability of the proband being group O is 0·5. If in fact he is group O the 'observed' score is 1, whereas if he is group A the 'observed' score is 0. The observed and expected scores are then summed and the difference compared statistically. The disadvantage of the method is that a great number of families are required for such analysis since many will be uninformative. For this reason the method has not been widely adopted.

Problems of disease association studies

Wiener (1970) has been particularly critical of studies of blood group associations but some of his criticisms are equally valid in *any* study of disease association. Excluding technical problems of erroneous typing and ambiguities in diagnosis and classification of disease, which should really not be problems in present day studies, the other main criticisms are largely concerned with the statistical treatment of the data.

Firstly, if a large enough number of different studies are made between a particular blood group and a particular disease then the results of 1 in 20 of these studies might appear 'significant' by chance alone. Or when studying many different HLA antigens for possible association with one particular disease one would expect that even if none of the antigens is really associated 1 out of 20 would appear associated by chance alone. This statistical problem is referred to as the Bonferroni inequality and Bodmer has suggested one answer to the problem is to multiply each P value obtained by the χ^2 test by the number of antigens tested, i.e. the number of comparisons. Thus with 20 comparisons an individual P value would have to be less than $0·05/20$ or 0·0025 to be significant. Better still the results of a pilot study should be confirmed by a more extensive prospective study.

Secondly, *prior* probabilities of their being an association are not taken into account. If diseases are selected at random and without clear rationale then the likelihood of an association may be remote. In such studies a P value of 0·05 would hardly be enough to overcome the presumption that no association exists. Unless there is a valid biological explanation for an observed association then perhaps a P value of 0·01 might be considered a more appropriate level of statistical significance.

Thirdly, in combining data from different centres there are a number of statistical problems perhaps the most important of which is pooling heterogeneous data.

Finally, there are the problems of 'stratification' and the choice of adequate controls. For example, there may be a stratum of the population in which both a particular disorder and blood group are especially frequent but with no causal connection between them. Controls must therefore be chosen from the same population as the patients. Also there is the possibility that healthy controls may be biased in favour of blood group O (Vogel, 1970).

With careful selection of controls and appropriate statistical analysis these problems can be avoided. However there remains the problem of the biological relevance of a blood group association. The strongest association is between duodenal ulcer and blood group O and non-secretor, yet even here the contribution of the ABO and secretor loci to the total variance is only about 2·5 per cent (Edwards, 1965). Thus the blood group loci would appear to contribute little to the genetic component of liability. However this seems unlikely to be the case with the HLA loci where the associations with certain diseases are very much stronger (McDevitt and Bodmer, 1974; Svejgaard *et al.*, 1975). The rather unrewarding results of studies of blood group associations should therefore not deter the investigator from considering disease associations with other marker traits, but always bearing in mind the importance of carefully selecting matched controls and the underlying problems of statistical analysis.

Value of disease association studies

There are a number of important practical reasons for studying disease associations. Firstly, an association with a genetic marker indicates an identifiable genetic component in the aetiology of the disorder. Possible explanations for blood group associations with various non-infectious and infectious diseases have been discussed respectively by Clarke (1961) and Vogel (1970). These associations are comparatively weak. However several associations which have recently been demonstrated with HLA antigens are much stronger (McDevitt and Bodmer, 1974; Svejgaard *et al.*, 1975). Some significant associations between various blood groups and HLA types are given in Tables 9.3 and 9.4. The figures for relative incidences are only approximate since they continually change as more studies are reported.

One of the most likely interpretations for the strong associations with HLA antigens is that immunological mechanisms, mediated by the HLA loci are involved in pathogenesis perhaps even by immunological cross-reaction between the HLA antigen and a possible aetiological agent(s). It could be that the homozygote for the particular HLA type may be at a higher risk of becoming affected or of manifesting a more severe form of the disease.

The identification of groups at risk through their HLA type (or other marker) may be useful in recognizing preclinical cases in families

Table 9.3 Significant associations between blood groups and disease

Disease	Blood group	Relative incidence (ave.)
Non-infectious		
Cancer of various sites	A	1·1–1·6
Pernicious anaemia	A	1·2
Ischaemic heart disease	A	1·2
Duodenal ulcer	O	1·3
Gastric ulcer	O	1·2
Infectious		
Leprosy	A	1·1
Hepatitis	A	1·3
Smallpox	A and AB	6·1
Influenza A₂	O	1·5

Table 9.4 Significant associations between HLA types and disease

Disease	HLA Antigen	Relative incidence (ave.)
Non-malignant		
Ankylosing spondylitis	B 27	135
Reiter's disease	B 27	45
Anterior uveitis	B 27	25
Coeliac disease	B 8	10
Myasthenia gravis	B 8	5
	A 2	
Multiple sclerosis	B 7	5
	A 3	1·8
Diabetes mellitus	B W 15	3
Malignant		
Hodgkins disease	B 18	1·9
	B 5	1·6
	A 1	1·4

where the marker trait is segregating and where a strong association has been demonstrated between the marker trait and the disorder in question. Clearly such information could be valuable in genetic counselling. For example, consider the risk to the children of an individual with ankylosing spondylitis. Family studies have shown that the empiric risk of the disease in first-degree relatives is about 4 per cent (higher in males than females). Further, the chance of having HLA antigen B 27 if one has ankylosing spondylitis is approximately 90 per cent whereas the proportion of healthy individuals with this HLA antigen is only about 5 per cent. If an affected parent has B 27 antigen and if a particular offspring is also found to have the B 27 antigen then the chances of its developing ankylosing spondylitis can be calculated to be of the order of 9 per cent. However if in this case the offspring is found *not* to have B 27 then the chances of its developing the disease is less than 1 per cent. Thus in this condition information on HLA typing may significantly affect the genetic advice one gives to relatives.

Finally when there is a strong association with a genetic marker this may be helpful in resolving genetic heterogeneity. For example myasthenia gravis may be a heterogeneous disorder because one form has been shown to be associated with HLA-B 8, has an early onset, and thymomas are uncommon. However another form is associated with HLA-A 2 and has a later onset and thymomas are commoner (Feltkamp *et al.*, 1974). These findings may have important practical implications as there is a suggestion that the two forms may respond differently to treatment by thymectomy (Fritze *et al.*, 1974). Therefore the resolution of heterogeneity by HLA typing may prove to have considerable practical importance in this disorder.

In conclusion, the study of disease associations has evolved over the last few years. Early studies on blood group associations, though not particularly rewarding, highlighted the importance of carefully choosing controls and applying the right statistical methods. The HLA system is without doubt the most polymorphic locus so far identified in man and therefore there is plenty of scope for studying possible disease associations. The recent demonstration of strong associations with certain HLA types is an exciting new development with important implications and should serve as a stimulus to search for other associations.

10. Parental Age and Birth Order

Probably the earliest report of a significant effect of parental age on the incidence of a genetic disorder was Sewall Wright's demonstration in 1926 of a maternal age effect in polydactyly and colour pattern in guinea pig (Wright, 1926). The rationale of studying parental age and birth order effects in human disorders and congenital malformations is that the results of such studies may throw some light on pathogenesis. Thus the demonstration of a parental age effect in sporadic cases of a chromosomal, autosomal dominant or X-linked disorder would indicate that mutation was related to parental age. Conversely in sporadic disorders of unknown aetiology where affected individuals do not reproduce, and so dominant inheritance cannot be proved, the demonstration of a parental age effect would suggest that such cases are perhaps due to fresh dominant mutations. In disorders not inherited in any simple manner (such as many congenital malformations) the demonstration of a parental age or birth order effect provides strong presumptive evidence of an environmental influence. Further, if the incidence of a disorder is shown to be related to parental age or birth order this information could be valuable for genetic counselling provided the effect is large enough. Such information is important in the derivation of empiric risks (p. 95).

So far the only abnormalities shown to be unequivocally related to *maternal* age are certain chromosomal disorders: trisomy-13 (Patau's syndrome), trisomy-18 (Edwards' syndrome) and trisomy-21 (Down's syndrome), and the XXX and XXY (Klinefelter's syndrome). On the other hand a number of unifactorial disorders have been shown to be related to *paternal* age. These include autosomal dominant disorders such as acrocephalosyndactyly (Apert's syndrome), achondroplasia, Marfan's syndrome, myositis ossificans, bilateral retinoblastoma and to a lesser extent some other dominant disorders (Jones et al., 1975). There is also evidence that paternal age may be a factor in new mutations in X-linked haemophilia A and perhaps Duchenne muscular dystrophy, in these cases the maternal grandfather's age being the important factor. Finally, certain sporadic disorders of unknown aetiology have also been shown to be related to paternal age, such as progeria and acrodysostosis (Jones et al., 1975).

Birth order effects have also been studied extensively (Carter, 1965). First born children are more often affected in congenital dislocation of the hip and to a lesser extent in congenital pyloric stenosis. On the other hand, haemolytic disease of the newborn is commoner in later born children, and whereas CNS malformations (anencephaly and spina bifida) are commonest in first born children the incidence rises again in high birth orders. In fact it seems that in CNS malformations among primiparae it is *younger* mothers who are at high risk, whereas among parities of three or more it is *older* mothers who are at greater risk (Fedrick, 1970).

In all such studies the main problem is disentangling the separate effects of maternal age, paternal age and birth order which are all correlated with each other. A number of statistical techniques have been developed for tackling this problem.

Method of Haldane and Smith

Haldane and Smith's (1947) method is perhaps the one most widely used for determining if there is a parental age or birth order effect. In this method the sum of the birth orders of all affected sibs (A) is compared with the theoretical value calculated on the assumption that there is no birth order effect. If A exceeds the theoretical value by more than about twice its standard error we may conclude that later born sibs are more likely to be affected, whereas if A is less than the theoretical value by more than twice its standard error then earlier born sibs are more often affected. The arithmetic is much simplified by testing $6A$ rather than A. Unclassified members of a sibship which occur only at the beginning or at the end of a sibship may be omitted. Thus if N denotes a normal sib, a an affected sib and '—' an unclassified sib, then a sibship—Na would be recorded as a sibship of size 2 with A equal to 2.

From knowing the total number of *classified* sibs (k) and affected sibs (h) in a sibship it is possible to determine the mean and variance of $6A$ from Table 10.2. A special case is when unclassified sibs do not occur at the beginning or end of a sibship. In such a case we have to calculate the mean and variance of $6A$.

The mean $= \dfrac{6hS_1}{k}$

and the variance

$$= \frac{36h(k - h)(kS_2 - S_1^2)}{k^2(k - 1)}$$

where h = number of affected sibs
k = number of classified sibs
S_1 = sum of the birth orders of all 'k' classified sibs
S_2 = sum of the *squares* of the birth orders for all 'k' classified sibs

Thus in a sibship $N - a$, the mean of $6A$

$$= \frac{(6)(1)(1 + 3)}{2}$$

$$= 12$$

and the variance of $6A$

$$= \frac{36(2 - 1)(2 \times 10 - 4^2)}{2^2(2 - 1)}$$

$$= 36$$

Having determined the birth order (A) and the mean and variance of $6A$ for each sibship, the data may then be tabulated as in the form given in Table 10.1, which in this case is based on data from 70 non-familial cases of adult onset myasthenia gravis, kindly made available by Dr Anne Jacob (Jacob, Clack and Emery, 1968). In this example the theoretical mean value is 1240 and its standard error is $\sqrt{6399 \cdot 50}$ or 80·0. The difference between the sum of $6A$ and the theoretical mean value is only 62 which is even less than the standard error. We may therefore conclude that in this disorder there is no significant parental age or birth order effect.

Table 10.1 Analysis of birth order in non-familial adult onset myasthenia gravis. N = normal; a = affected; — = unclassified; k = number of classified sibs; h = number of affected sibs; A = birth order.

Family no.	Sibship	k	h	A	$6A$	Mean	Variance
1	aN	2	1	1	6	9	9
2	N———NaN	4	1	6	36	28·5	186·75
3	a	1	1	1	6	6	0
4	NaN	3	1	2	12	12	24
5	aN	2	1	1	6	9	9
6	aNNNNNNNN	9	1	1	6	30	240
7	NNNaNNNN	8	1	4	24	27	189
*8	——NNNNaNN	7	1	5	30	24	144
.							
.							
.							
.							
.							
.							
70	NNNNa	5	1	5	30	18	72
	Total	330	70	217	1302	1240	6399·50

* Unclassified sibs omitted.

Though this test is easy to apply it does not answer the question whether it is maternal age, paternal age, birth order or a combination

Table 10.2 Mean (black figures) and Variance (ordinary figures) of $6A$ in complete sibships. k = number of classified sibs; h = number of affected sibs. (*From* Haldane and Smith, 1947)

k \ h	1	2	3	4	5	6	7	8	9	10	11	12	13	14	15	16	17	18	19
2	**9**	**18**	—	—	—	—	—	—	—	—	—	—	—	—	—	—	—	—	—
	9	0																	
3	**12**	**24**	**36**	—	—	—	—	—	—	—	—	—	—	—	—	—	—	—	—
	24	24	0																
4	**15**	**30**	**45**	**60**	—	—	—	—	—	—	—	—	—	—	—	—	—	—	—
	45	60	45	0															
5	**18**	**36**	**54**	**72**	**90**	—	—	—	—	—	—	—	—	—	—	—	—	—	—
	72	108	108	72	0														
6	**21**	**42**	**63**	**84**	**105**	**126**	—	—	—	—	—	—	—	—	—	—	—	—	—
	105	168	189	168	105	0													
7	**24**	**48**	**72**	**96**	**120**	**144**	**168**	—	—	—	—	—	—	—	—	—	—	—	—
	144	240	288	288	240	144	0												
8	**27**	**54**	**81**	**108**	**135**	**162**	**189**	**216**	—	—	—	—	—	—	—	—	—	—	—
	189	324	405	432	405	324	189	0											
9	**30**	**60**	**90**	**120**	**150**	**180**	**210**	**240**	**270**	—	—	—	—	—	—	—	—	—	—
	240	420	540	600	600	540	420	240	0										
10	**33**	**66**	**99**	**132**	**165**	**198**	**231**	**264**	**297**	**330**	—	—	—	—	—	—	—	—	—
	297	528	693	792	825	792	693	528	297	0									

Table 10.2—continued

k	h	1	2	3	4	5	6	7	8	9	10	11	12	13	14	15	16	17	18	19
11		36	72	108	144	180	216	252	288	324	360	396	—							
		360	648	864	1008	1080	1080	1008	864	648	360	0								
12		39	78	117	156	195	234	273	312	351	390	429	468							
		429	780	1053	1248	1365	1404	1365	1248	1053	780	429	0							
13		42	84	126	168	210	252	294	336	378	420	462	504	546						
		504	924	1260	1512	1680	1764	1764	1680	1512	1260	924	504	0						
14		45	90	135	180	225	270	315	360	405	450	495	540	585	630					
		585	1080	1485	1800	2025	2160	2205	2160	2025	1800	1485	1080	585	0					
15		48	96	144	192	240	288	336	384	432	480	528	576	624	672	720				
		672	1248	1728	2112	2400	2592	2688	2688	2592	2400	2112	1728	1248	672	0				
16		51	102	153	204	255	306	357	408	459	510	561	612	663	714	765	816			
		765	1428	1989	2448	2805	3060	3213	3264	3213	3060	2805	2448	1989	1428	765	0			
17		54	108	162	216	270	324	378	432	486	540	594	648	702	756	810	864	918		
		864	1620	2268	2808	3240	3564	3780	3888	3888	3780	3564	3240	2808	2268	1620	864	0		
18		57	114	171	228	285	342	399	456	513	570	627	684	741	798	855	912	969	1026	
		969	1824	2565	3192	3705	4104	4389	4560	4617	4560	4389	4104	3705	3192	2565	1824	969	0	
19		60	120	180	240	300	360	420	480	540	600	660	720	780	840	900	960	1020	1080	1140
		1080	2040	2880	3600	4200	4680	5040	5280	5400	5400	5280	5040	4680	4200	3600	2880	2040	1080	0
20		63	126	189	252	315	378	441	504	567	630	693	756	819	882	945	1008	1071	1134	1197
		1197	2268	3213	4032	4725	5292	5733	6048	6237	6300	6237	6048	5733	5292	4725	4032	3213	2268	1197

of these factors which is important. Other methods have to be used to determine the separate effects of these various factors. Further, this test will not be informative if the disorder in question is associated with *both* early and late pregnancies, these two effects tending to cancel each other out. If such a situation is a possibility then the method of Barton and David (1958) may be used to resolve the problem.

Choice of controls

The simplest way of demonstrating a parental age or birth order effect is to make comparisons with the birth of unaffected sibs. However this assumes that the disorder in question is not likely to affect the parents' decision to have further children. A serious disorder present at birth or with onset in childhood may well deter some parents from having further children. In such a situation the use of normal sibs as controls would result in an apparent greater parental age and birth order. This method is therefore only justified in the case of disorders with onset in adulthood.

An alternative approach is to make comparisons with a sample of control families in which the disorder in question does not occur. But here the difficulty is to choose as controls parents who are truly comparable to the parents of affected individuals. This is notoriously difficult.

A simple method which has often been used and which avoids some of these difficulties is to compare maternal age, paternal age and birth order in a series of families with comparable data from the general population. This has been done for example in Apert's syndrome (Blank, 1960), myositis ossificans (Tünte, Becker and Knorre, 1967), achondroplasia (Murdoch *et al.*, 1970) and Marfan's syndrome (Murdoch, Walker and McKusick, 1972). Some population data on parental age and birth order in three different countries are given in Table 10.3. Unfortunately in Britain population statistics for paternal age were not available before 1962. However on the basis of studies over a number of years of a large series of births in England and Wales, Fraser and Friedmann (1967) have calculated that between 1900 to 1962 the mean difference between paternal and maternal ages at the birth of a child was about 3·1 years. Therefore for this period an approximate estimate of paternal age can be derived from maternal age by adding 3·1 years. Bundey and her colleagues (1975) have derived more accurate estimates of paternal age by determining the appropriate age difference between spouses *according to the mother's age,* since this difference is not the same for all maternal ages, and then adding this difference to maternal age. Armed with such information one may then compare not only the mean parental ages in patients' families with those expected, but also the mean *differences* between parental ages in patients' families with those expected.

Table 10.3 Population data on parental age and birth order

Source	Maternal age Mean	s.d.	Paternal age Mean	s.d.	Birth order Mean	s.d.
England and Wales, 1950 (Blank, 1960)	28·04	5·97	—	—	2·24	1·57
London, 1960 (Blank, 1960)	—	—	31·69	6·47	1·86	1·21
*England and Wales, 1973	25·79	5·10	28·58	6·13	1·95	1·16
Australia, 1953 (Blank, 1960)	27·65	5·84	31·04	6·79	—	—
United States, 1955 (Murdoch et al., 1970)	26·54	6·07	29·85	6·95	2·64	1·73

* Calculated from data in Registrar General (1975) *Statistical Review of England and Wales for the year 1973, Part 2.* HMSO, London.

It should be noted that in making such comparisons with the general population secular changes in parental ages over the years covered by the births of affected individuals being studied must be taken into account. Comparisons should therefore be made with controls of roughly the *same period of time* and from a *similar environment*. In

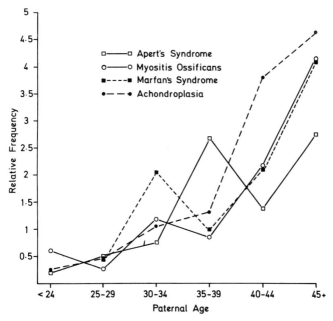

Fig. 10.1 Number of fathers of affected offspring relative to the number in the general population in various age groups (calculated from the original data).

Table 10.4 are given data on parental ages and birth order calculated from information in the Registrar General's Reports for England and Wales from 1940 to 1973.

Table 10.4 Parental age and birth order in England and Wales calculated from information in the Registrar General's Reports for 1940 to 1973

Year	Maternal age Mean	s.d.	Paternal age Mean	s.d.	Birth order Mean	s.d.
1940	28·53	5·98	—	—	2·37	1·90
1941	28·55	6·06	—	—	2·36	1·91
1942	28·66	5·99	—	—	2·25	1·81
1943	28·84	6·06	—	—	2·21	1·75
1944	29·06	6·09	—	—	2·26	1·68
1945	29·12	6·19	—	—	2·27	1·69
1946	29·01	5·91	—	—	2·16	1·59
1947	28·54	5·90	—	—	2·09	1·53
1948	28·26	5·99	—	—	2·15	1·56
1949	28·03	5·94	—	—	2·16	1·54
1950	28·04	5·97	—	—	2·24	1·57
1951	28·02	5·89	—	—	2·22	1·54
1952	27·79	5·81	—	—	2·24	1·56
1953	27·70	5·74	—	—	2·23	1·54
1954	27·62	5·75	—	—	2·23	1·54
1955	27·57	5·75	—	—	2·23	1·54
1956	27·46	5·75	—	—	2·22	1·53
1957	27·40	5·75	—	—	2·22	1·53
1958	27·30	5·73	—	—	2·22	1·52
1959	27·22	5·73	—	—	2·24	1·53
1960	27·20	5·77	—	—	2·27	1·53
1961	27·09	5·80	30·17	6·68	2·28	1·54
1962	26·96	5·80	30·04	6·66	2·29	1·54
1963	26·87	5·77	29·93	6·62	2·31	1·54
1964	26·80	5·77	29·85	6·62	2·32	1·53
1965	26·63	5·77	29·67	6·64	2·27	1·49
1966	26·38	5·74	29·42	6·64	2·24	1·47
1967	26·26	5·69	29·27	6·63	2·20	1·43
1968	26·13	5·59	29·11	6·56	2·18	1·40
1969	26·02	5·51	28·94	6·50	2·14	1·36
1970	25·87	5·41	28·75	6·42	2·11	1·31
1971	25·78	5·32	28·60	6·35	2·06	1·27
1972	25·78	5·22	28·59	6·25	2·01	1·22
1973	25·79	5·10	28·58	6·13	1·95	1·16

A simple and effective graphical way of demonstrating a parental age effect is to determine for each age group the number of parents of affected individuals relative to the number in the general population (Fig. 10.1). A five-year interval size is useful for this purpose.

To determine if there is any significant difference between the mean ages of parents and controls one may use the 'Student's' t test. If a *large* general population is being used for comparison then

$$t = \frac{m - \mu}{s/\sqrt{n}}$$

where m = mean parental age in the sample
s = standard deviation of parental age in the sample
n = number of fathers or mothers in the sample
μ = mean parental age in the general population

Thus in a study of Marfan's syndrome (Murdoch *et al.*, 1972) the mean maternal age of 23 sporadic cases was 29·30 (s.d. 5·36) compared with the mean maternal age in the general population of 26·54 (s.d. 6·07), i.e. a difference of 2·76 years.

Therefore
$$t = \frac{29·30 - 26·54}{5·36/\sqrt{23}}$$

$$= 2·5$$

With $(n - 1)$ degrees of freedom, i.e. 22, from Tables of 'Student's' t distribution $P = 0·02$, and therefore the mean age of mothers at the birth of offspring with Marfan's syndrome is significantly greater than in the general population. In this study however, the mean paternal age was 36·61 (s.d. 9·06) compared with a mean paternal age in the general population of 29·85 (s.d. 6·95). Here the difference is 6·76 years which is highly significant ($P < 0·01$). Thus paternal age is elevated more than maternal age but in fact both are significantly greater than the general population.

Birth order is not normally distributed and therefore it is not statistically legitimate to make comparisons in this way. Further, this approach is limited in distinguishing the separate effects of parental age and birth order. The so-called *Greenwood-Yule Method* (Greenwood and Yule, 1914), subsequently modified by McKeown and Record (1956), was developed in order to separate the effects of maternal age and birth order but the method does not take into account paternal age. To evaluate separately these various factors the method of partial correlations is usually used.

Method of partial correlations

This method has been widely used in determining the separate effects of paternal age, maternal age and birth order (Penrose, 1957), though it has to be recognized that it may not be statistically entirely satisfactory (Smith, C. A. B., 1972).

Essentially the method allows one to compare the effect of a single variable on incidence while other variables are held constant. For example, to estimate the effect of paternal age on incidence while maternal age and birth order are held constant. In statistics wherever there are more than two variables and a correlation between any pair is to be determined, the effect of one or more of the remaining variables being eliminated (held constant), this is referred to as a *partial correlation coefficient*. Thus if there are four variables represented as 1, 2, 3 and 4, then we first determine the usual (product-moment) correlation between each pair of variables: r_{12}, r_{13}, r_{23}, etc. The partial correlation between any pair of variables (e.g. incidence and maternal age, paternal age or birth order) eliminating the other two variables can then be calculated. Thus between 1 and 2 eliminating 3 and 4 (written as $r_{12 \cdot 34}$) by

$$r_{12 \cdot 34} = \frac{r_{12 \cdot 4} - r_{13 \cdot 4} r_{23 \cdot 4}}{\sqrt{(1 - r_{13 \cdot 4}^2)(1 - r_{23 \cdot 4}^2)}}$$

where coefficients like $r_{12 \cdot 4}$ can be calculated by

$$r_{12 \cdot 4} = \frac{r_{12} - r_{14} r_{24}}{\sqrt{(1 - r_{14}^2)(1 - r_{24}^2)}}$$

In practice, to determine the independent effects of parental age and birth order we calculate the following correlations:

A   From population data (see Table 10.5)
    1. Paternal age and maternal age   : r_{PM}
    2. Paternal age and birth order   : r_{PA}
    3. Maternal age and birth order   : r_{MA}

B   From the families being studied
    4. Paternal age and disease incidence   : r_{PI}
    5. Maternal age and disease incidence   : r_{MI}
    6. Birth order and disease incidence   : r_{AI}

and from these we derive the partial correlations between

    7. Paternal age and disease incidence, maternal age
        and birth order being eliminated   : $r_{PI \cdot MA}$
    8. Maternal age and disease incidence, paternal age
        and birth order being eliminated   : $r_{MI \cdot PA}$
    9. Birth order and disease incidence, paternal age and
        maternal age being eliminated   : $r_{AI \cdot PM}$

Table 10.5 Correlations from various population studies

	Source	Correlation	Reference
Paternal and maternal age	Australia (1953)	0·73	Blank (1960)
	USA (1955)	0·76	Murdoch et al. (1970)
	England and Wales (1973)	0·72	Unpublished*
	Scotland (1973)	0·77	Unpublished*
Paternal age and birth order	London (1960)	0·30	Blank (1960)
Maternal age and birth order	England and Wales (1950)	0·49	Blank (1960)
	USA (1955)	0·52	Murdoch et al (1970)
	England and Wales (1973)	0·45	Unpublished*
	Scotland (1973)	0·49	Unpublished*

* Calculated from data in: Registrar General (1975) *Statistical Review of England and Wales for the year 1973.* Part 2. London: H.M.S.O. Registrar General, Scotland (1974) *Annual Report for 1973,* Parts 1 + 2. Edinburgh: H.M.S.O.

The partial correlation between paternal age and disease incidence, birth order being eliminated, is

$$r_{PI\,.\,A} = \frac{r_{PI} - r_{PA}r_{IA}}{\sqrt{(1 - r_{PA}^2)(1 - r_{IA}^2)}}$$

and between paternal age and maternal age, birth order being eliminated, is

$$r_{PM\,.\,A} = \frac{r_{PM} - r_{PA}r_{MA}}{\sqrt{(1 - r_{PA}^2)(1 - r_{MA}^2)}}$$

and between maternal age and disease incidence, birth order being eliminated, is

$$r_{MI\,.\,A} = \frac{r_{MI} - r_{MA}r_{IA}}{\sqrt{(1 - r_{MA}^2)(1 - r_{IA}^2)}}$$

and so on. From these partial correlation coefficients we can then calculate the partial correlation between paternal age and disease incidence, maternal age *and* birth order being eliminated:

$$r_{PI\,.\,MA} = \frac{r_{PI\,.\,A} - r_{PM\,.\,A}r_{MI\,.\,A}}{\sqrt{(1 - r_{PM\,.\,A}^2)(1 - r_{MI\,.\,A}^2)}}$$

Thus in Blank's study of Apert's syndrome (Blank, 1960):

from population data

$$r_{PM} = 0\cdot73$$

$$r_{PA} = 0\cdot30$$

$$r_{MA} = 0\cdot49$$

from the families being studied

$$r_{PI} = 0\cdot34$$

$$r_{MI} = 0\cdot31$$

$$r_{AI} = 0\cdot14$$

Therefore

$$r_{PI\,.\,M} = \frac{0\cdot34 - (0\cdot73)(0\cdot31)}{\sqrt{(1 - 0\cdot73^2)(1 - 0\cdot31^2)}}$$

$$= 0\cdot18$$

Similarly

$$r_{PI\,.\,A} = 0\cdot32, \quad r_{MI\,.\,P} = 0\cdot10, \quad r_{MI\,.\,A} = 0\cdot28,$$

$$r_{AI\,.\,P} = 0\cdot04, \quad r_{AI\,.\,M} = -0\cdot01, \quad \text{and} \quad r_{PM\,.\,A} = 0\cdot70$$

Finally the partial correlation between paternal age and disease incidence, maternal age and birth order being eliminated, is calculated

$$r_{PI\,.\,MA} = \frac{0\cdot32 - (0\cdot70)(0\cdot28)}{\sqrt{(1 - 0\cdot70^2)(1 - 0\cdot28^2)}}$$

$$= 0\cdot18$$

Similarly

$$r_{MI\,.\,PA} = 0\cdot09 \quad \text{and} \quad r_{AI\,.\,PM} = 0\cdot00$$

Therefore paternal age is the main factor because when maternal age and birth order are eliminated there remains a positive partial correlation of 0·18 between paternal age and disease incidence. On the other hand when paternal age and birth order are eliminated then the correlation between maternal age and disease incidence is only 0·09, and there is no correlation between birth order and disease incidence when paternal and maternal age are eliminated.

In all these calculations it is necessary to re-emphasise a word of caution in using population data on parental ages or correlations between parental ages and birth order. The general population with which comparisons are being made must be similar to the parents being studied both in time and place since these parameters are known to be affected by a variety of socio-economic factors.

The significance of an ordinary correlation coefficient, for a relatively small sample size (as is the case in most family studies), may be determined from Tables (Appendix 3, p. 133) or by calculating 'Student's' t which for an ordinary correlation coefficient is

$$= \frac{r\sqrt{n-2}}{\sqrt{1-r^2}}$$

with $(n-2)$ degrees of freedom. In the case of a partial correlation coefficient where two variables have been eliminated 'Student's' t is

$$= \frac{r\sqrt{n-4}}{\sqrt{1-r^2}}$$

with $(n-4)$ degrees of freedom. The significance of t values can be determined from Tables (Appendix 1, p. 131).

In order to determine if two correlation coefficients differ significantly they are first transformed to so-called 'z' values where:

$$z_1 = \tfrac{1}{2} \log_e \frac{1+r_1}{1-r_1}$$

and

$$z_2 = \tfrac{1}{2} \log_e \frac{1+r_2}{1-r_2}$$

Fortunately there are Tables (see Appendix 4, p. 134) for transforming 'r' values into 'z' values. We can then calculate the normal deviate:

$$x = \frac{|z_1 - z_2|}{\sqrt{\dfrac{1}{n_1 - 3} + \dfrac{1}{n_2 - 3}}}$$

If the second sample represents the general population, and therefore n_2 is very large, then the normal deviate becomes:

$$\frac{|z_1 - z_2|}{\sqrt{\dfrac{1}{n_1 - 3}}}$$

We can then determine if the difference is significant from tables (p. 122).

Partial correlation coefficients may be compared in the same way as ordinary (product-moment) correlation coefficients except that in the above formulae 'n' is replaced by n minus as many variables as have been eliminated from the comparison in question. Thus if we were comparing the partial correlation coefficients of paternal age and disease incidence with maternal age and disease incidence, in each case eliminating birth order and the other parental age, then the normal deviate would be:

$$\frac{|z_1 - z_2|}{\sqrt{\dfrac{1}{n_1 - 5} + \dfrac{1}{n_2 - 5}}}$$

In conclusion, proving that a parental age or birth order effect on disease incidence exists, if not obvious on casual inspection of family data, may be difficult. The method of partial correlations is relatively simple to apply but it may not be statistically entirely satisfactory though it can be used to give at least a first approximation. Probably the best method of estimating the separate effects of maternal age, paternal age and birth order is by *multiple regression analysis* (Smith, C. A. B., 1972) but the method is complex and outside the scope of this book.

Should a parental age or birth order effect be demonstrated this should not be regarded as the end of an investigation. It is rather the beginning of an enquiry since it may suggest possible lines for further research. In the case of a congenital malformation of unknown aetiology it suggests the importance of environmental factors in causation which should then be sought for in relation to parental age and/or birth order.

Thus persistent patent ductus arteriosus is commoner in first borns. Now the normal closure of the ductus shortly after birth depends upon adequate oxygenation of the blood. Since difficulties in labour, with possible resultant fetal anoxia, are commoner in first pregnancies than in later pregnancies this may be the explanation for the birth order effect in this abnormality. In fact the incidence of fetal distress is higher among affecteds than would be expected.

Finally if the effect is sufficiently marked information on parental age and birth order may also be used to construct risk tables for use in genetic counselling as in the case of Down's syndrome and maternal age.

11. Recognition and Estimation of Changes in Disease Frequency

In studying the possible relevance of environmental factors in the aetiology of say a particular congenital malformation, one approach to the problem is to study changes in frequency over time. If there is a dramatic change at a particular point in time one would then attempt to identify the environmental factor which caused this change. Such a change might be recognized by an astute observer without recourse to statistical techniques. An outstanding example of this was the recognition by Lenz in Germany and McBride in Australia of the teratogenic effects of thalidomide, a drug which first appeared on the market as a sedative in the late 1950s. During 1961, Lenz (1961) and McBride (1961) reported that they were seeing many more cases of a rare form of limb deformity (a type of phocomelia) than had been their previous experience. On taking a careful history they discovered that the mothers of these children had all taken the drug thalidomide in early pregnancy. This approach, however, is not possible with relatively common disorders because a very large number of cases would be needed to detect any significant change in frequency. In such situations we have to rely on statistical methods.

Incidence and prevalence

So far, for the sake of simplicity, we have usually referred to the number of cases of a disorder in a population as its *frequency*. There are, however, two estimates of frequency which are not necessarily identical. *Incidence* refers to the number of *new* cases per unit of population. For example, the incidence of Down's syndrome is 1·4 per 1000 live births or about 1 in 700 live births. *Prevalence* on the other hand refers to *all* cases present in a population, either within a given period (so-called *period* prevalence rate) or a particular point in time (so-called *point* prevalence rate), per unit of population at risk at that time. In the case of Down's syndrome prevalence is much less than incidence because of early mortality in this condition. In the case of congenital malformations incidence is more precisely known than prevalence, the latter being notoriously unreliable.

Comparison of proportions

If we wish to determine if there has been a significant change in the frequency (incidence or prevalence) of a particular disorder we could merely compare the proportion of cases in one year with the proportion in another using standard statistical techniques.

Thus if the proportion of cases (P_1) in the first period was

$$n_1/N_1$$

and in the second period (P_2) was

$$n_2/N_2$$

and if

$$P_0 = \frac{n_1 + n_2}{N_1 + N_2}$$

Then in the usual manner (see Snedecor and Cochran, 1967) we can calculate 'x' the so-called normal deviate where

$$x = \frac{|P_1 - P_2|}{\sqrt{P_0(1 - P_0)(1/N_1 + 1/N_2)}}$$

(The vertical lines $|P_1 - P_2|$ mean that we subtract whichever is the smaller from the larger of the proportions.) If the sample size (N) is relatively small (say less than 200) then in such calculations a *correction for continuity* may be included. Details are to be found in most standard statistical texts. If the value of 'x' exceeds 1·96 then the proportions differ significantly ($P = 0.05$). The exact level of significance of 'x' can be determined from tables of the normal distribution (Fisher and Yates, 1963). The points most commonly required for significance are given in Table 11.1.

Table 11.1   Probability (P) of deviations (x) in units of standard deviation from the mean assuming normal distribution.

P	0·20	0·10	0·05	0·02	0·01	0·002	0·001	0·0001
x	1·28	1·65	1·96	2·33	2·58	3·09	3·29	3·89

It should be noted that $x^2 = \chi^2$ and the same results may be obtained by presenting the data in a 2×2 table and determining the significance of the χ^2 value with 1 degree of freedom. The calculation, however, is more laborious than using proportions.

The method of calculation is illustrated with data on the incidence of CNS malformations (anencephaly and spina bifida) in the Edinburgh region. For several years the incidence of these malformations had remained fairly steady at about 1 in 200 total (still and live) births. However in 1971 there appeared to be an increase in the incidence to 1 in 120 births and the question arises as to whether this figure is

significantly different from previous years. The actual figures were 50
CNS malformations out of 9706 total births in 1970, and 79 out of
9771 births in 1971. Thus:

for 1970

$$P_1 = \frac{50}{9706}$$

$$= 0{\cdot}0052$$

for 1971

$$P_2 = \frac{79}{9771}$$

$$= 0{\cdot}0081$$

and

$$P_0 = \frac{50 + 79}{9706 + 9771}$$

$$= 0{\cdot}0066$$

and

$$x = \frac{|P_1 - P_2|}{\sqrt{P_0(1 - P_0)(1/N_1 + 1/N_2)}}$$

$$= \frac{(0{\cdot}0081 - 0{\cdot}0052)}{\sqrt{(0{\cdot}0066)(0{\cdot}9934)(1/9706 + 1/9771)}}$$

$$= 2{\cdot}5$$

Thus the difference in proportions is statistically significant ($P < 0{\cdot}02$).
In subsequent years the incidence returned again to about 1 in 200
births and no satisfactory explanation could be found for the increase
in 1971.

The method is only applicable if n_1 and n_2 are reasonably large (say
more than 20). Further, when many comparisons are made a number
of differences may turn out to appear significant by chance alone (i.e.
1 in 20).

Another approach is to consider an overall significance test using
a $2 \times k$ contingency table and determine whether there is a significant
trend in the proportions from Group 1 to Group k (Armitage, 1955).
However the method of calculation is somewhat tedious and does not
have the immediate visual appeal of the so-called cumulative sum or
cusum techniques.

Cumulative sum techniques

These techniques (Woodward and Goldsmith, 1964) were originally
developed for use in industry to demonstrate phenomena such as trends

in productivity, but they can also be used to pinpoint the onset of an epidemic or an increase in the incidence of a particular congenital malformation.

The basic procedure merely consists of subtracting a previously defined 'reference value' (k) from each number in the series and accumulating the sum of the differences as each additional figure is introduced. The successive accumulated differences are referred to as the 'cumulative sums' (*cusums*) and the graph of these sums is known as the 'cumulative sum chart'. Thus if the individual numbers of cases in successive years are

$$n_1, n_2, n_3, \ldots n_r,$$

then

$$S_1 = (n_1 - k)$$
$$S_2 = (n_1 - k) + (n_2 - k) = S_1 + (n_2 - k)$$
$$S_3 = S_2 + (n_3 - k)$$

and $\qquad S_r = S_{r-1} + (n_r - k) = n_1 + n_2 + \ldots n_r - rk$

The reference value is chosen as the number around which the results are expected to vary, usually the mean value of the results at the beginning of a period of study. To simplify the calculation of cusums, 'k' is suitably rounded off. If the average of the results is close to the reference value, some of the differences will be positive and some negative so that the cusum chart will be essentially horizontal. However, if the average begins to rise more of the differences will become positive and the cusum chart will slope upwards.

The value of the technique is illustrated in the following example. Suppose the annual incidence (say number per 10 000 births suitably rounded to the nearest whole number for convenience) of a particular congenital malformation is as given in Table 11.2. If the annual incidence is plotted there is no clear trend or change over the period of study (Fig. 11.1). However, if the cusums are calculated with $k = 20$ (Table 11.2), and plotted (Fig. 11.1) it becomes clear that the annual incidence began to rise in 1967. The average incidence during the period 1950 to 1966 was about 21. The importance of choosing a reference value close to this is illustrated in Figure 11.2. If too low a value is chosen the cusum plot increases steadily throughout whereas if too high a value is chosen all the cusums are negative.

If the method is applied to absolute *numbers* of cases, then in an expanding population the number of cases would automatically increase, and be reflected by a change in cusums, even if the relative incidence remained the same. The method is therefore best applied to *incidence rates* (e.g. number per 10 000 births) as in the above example.

It should be noted that this method is essentially merely a graphical

Table 11.2   Annual incidence and cusums ($k = 20$)

Year	Incidence	Difference from k	Cusums
1950	22	+2	2
1951	29	+9	11
1952	28	+8	19
1953	23	+3	22
1954	9	−11	11
1955	28	+8	19
1956	12	−8	11
1957	30	+10	21
1958	14	−6	15
1959	28	+8	23
1960	15	−5	18
1961	18	−2	16
1962	27	+7	23
1963	9	−11	12
1964	30	+10	22
1965	14	−6	16
1966	24	+4	20
1967	27	+7	27
1968	30	+10	37
1969	15	−5	32
1970	29	+9	41
1971	26	+6	47
1972	30	+10	57
1973	26	+6	63
1974	19	−1	62
1975	32	+12	74

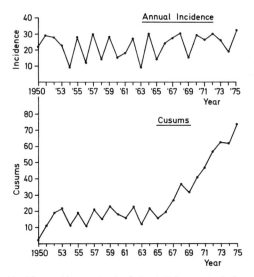

Fig. 11.1 Annual incidence. Above: standard chart. Below: cumulative sum chart. (Data from Table 11.2.)

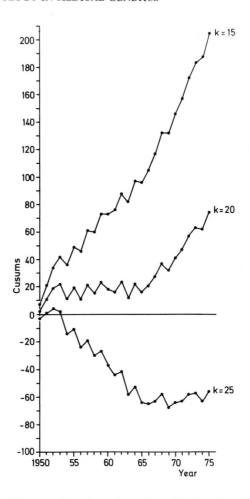

Fig. 11.2 Cumulative sum charts for various values of k. (Data from Table 11.2.)

means of demonstrating a change. If the reader wishes to define such a change in precise terms then it is best to apply one of the more conventional statistical methods which are available for this purpose (e.g. *see* Armitage, 1971).

Cyclical changes

There are a number of disorders which show seasonal variations or cyclical trends in incidence, for example, hay fever is without doubt seasonal with the highest incidence in summer months. The demonstration of a seasonal variation in incidence for a particular disorder or congenital malformation would indicate that environmental factors are involved and thus give a clue to aetiology. For this reason a number of studies in recent years have been directed to this problem. A commonly used method of demonstrating seasonal variation is to compare the observed incidence with the expected incidence using a simple χ^2 test. Using this method, for example, Nielsen, Holm and Haahr (1975) showed that there was a significant seasonal variation in the birth of children with sex chromosomal abnormalities with the highest incidences occurring in March, April and May. However, this is not a good test for detecting cyclical trends for reasons which have been discussed by Edwards (1961). Further, considerable difficulty can be experienced in attempting to demonstrate a cyclical trend which is not apparent on casual inspection of the data.

Edwards (1961) has developed a very ingenious statistical technique for recognizing and estimating cyclical trends and this has recently been further developed by Walter and Elwood (1975). Essentially the method consists of estimating the amplitude of seasonal variations and the time at which the maximum occurs in a postulated simple harmonic fluctuation. These methods are best used when the sample size is large, that is, when the total number of events (e.g. congenital malformations) in one year exceeds 50. However, the method of calculation is complicated and really requires a computer programme for analysis.

A much simpler ranking (non-parametric) method has been introduced by Hewitt et al. (1971) which is particularly valuable for sample sizes less than 50 provided that at least 6 of the 12 months must have non-zero frequencies. The method first consists of ranking the incidence rates for each month, the highest incidence as 12 and the lowest as unity. The next step is to decide if there is a prior hypothesis for specifying a six month period of higher expected incidences, or if the likely nature of any seasonal variation has to be inferred from the data. In the latter case when no prior hypothesis exists it is necessary to determine the six month period which yields the highest value of the rank-sum. With a pre-assigned six month period a rank-sum equal to or greater than 50 would be significant whereas for *any* six month period a rank-sum equal to or greater than 55 is required for significance (Table 11.3).

A six month period is chosen for these calculations because the chance probability of obtaining the largest possible rank-sum is smallest for this period (Hewitt et al., 1971).

The method of calculation is illustrated with data on the monthly incidence of anencephaly (still births) among total births in Scotland for the five year period 1969 to 1973 (*Registrar General Scotland, Annual Reports for 1969 to 1973*). Inspection of the data suggests a seasonal variation with most births occurring in the winter months (Table 11.4). The maximum rank-sum is from September to February and amounts

Table 11.3 Cumulative probabilities of various rank-sums for pre-assigned six month periods or for any six month period. (*From* Hewitt *et al.*, 1971)

Rank-sum	Cumulative probabilities	
	Pre-assigned 6 month period	Any 6 month period
57	0·0011	0·0134
56	0·0022	0·0248
55	0·0043	0·0464
54	0·0076	0·0766
53	0·0130	0·1260
52	0·0206	0·1914
51	0·0325	0·2908
50	0·0465	0·3826
49	0·0660	0·4958·
48	0·0898	0·6086
47	0·1201	0·7258
46	0·1548	0·8310
45	0·1970	0·9138
44	0·2424	0·9614
43	0·2944	0·9904
42	0·3496	0·9986
41	0·4091	1·0000
40	0·4686	—
39 or less	1·0000	—

to 56 which according to Table 11.3 is statistically significant with $P = 0.0248$.

The relative merits of the various tests devised by Edwards (1961), Walter and Elwood (1975) and Hewitt *et al.* (1971) for studying cyclical changes are discussed by Walter and Elwood (1975). In general

Table 11.4 Seasonal variation in the incidence of anencephaly in Scotland from 1969 to 1973 inclusive

Month of birth	Total births	Anencephalics		Rank	Maximum rank
		No.	Incidence/1000		
January	34 110	94	2·76	10	10
February	30 840	93	3·02	12	12
March	35 400	69	1·95	3	—
April	32 548	79	2·43	7	—
May	33 635	64	1·90	2	—
June	32 523	71	2·18	5	—
July	33 037	67	2·03	4	—
August	32 115	56	1·74	1	—
September	30 791	79	2·57	9	9
October	33 365	83	2·49	8	8
November	29 565	82	2·77	11	11
December	31 304	74	2·36	6	6
				Rank-sum	56

whenever the sample size is small (N < 50) then a non-parametric method is preferable. But this method will only detect a fairly marked and consistent seasonal variation. A parametric method is preferable when there is a substantial amount of data.

It should always be borne in mind, of course, that in studying a particular disorder or congenital malformation the demonstration of a significant change in incidence, which may or may not be cyclical, is not an end in itself but merely the first step in attempting to identify possible aetiological factors.

Appendices

1. 'Student's' t-distribution
2. χ^2 Distribution
3. Correlation coefficient
4. Transformation of r to z
5. Normal distribution for estimation of h^2
6. Lod scores

Appendices 1, 2 and 3 are from Bailey, N. T. J. (1969) *Statistical Methods in Biology*. London: English Universities Press; Appendix 4 from *Introduction to Biostatistics* by Robert R. Sokal and F. James Rohlf, W. H. Freeman and Company © 1973; Appendix 5 from Falconer, D. S. (1965) *Annals of Human Genetics* (*London*) **29,** 51–76 and Appendix 6 calculated from Smith, C. A. B. (1968) *Annals of Human Genetics* (*London*), **32,** 127–50, with some additional values specially made available by Professor C. A. B. Smith.

Appendix 1. 'Student's' t-distribution.
The table gives the percentage points most frequently required for significance tests and confidence limits based on 'Student's' t-distribution. Thus the probability of observing a value of t, with 10 degrees of freedom, greater in *absolute value* than 3·169 (i.e. < −3·169 or > +3·169) is exactly 0·01 or 1 per cent.

Degrees of freedom	Value of P					
	0·10	0·05	0·02	0·01	0·002	0·001
1	6·314	12·71	31·82	63·66	318·3	636·6
2	2·920	4·303	6·965	9·925	22·33	31·60
3	2·353	3·182	4·541	5·841	10·21	12·92
4	2·132	2·776	3·747	4·604	7·173	8·610
5	2·015	2·571	3·365	4·032	5·893	6·869
6	1·943	2·447	3·143	3·707	5·208	5·959
7	1·895	2·365	2·998	3·499	4·785	5·408
8	1·860	2·306	2·896	3·355	4·501	5·041
9	1·833	2·262	2·821	3·250	4·297	4·781
10	1·812	2·228	2·764	3·169	4·144	4·587
11	1·796	2·201	2·718	3·106	4·025	4·437
12	1·782	2·179	2·681	3·055	3·930	4·318
13	1·771	2·160	2·650	3·012	3·852	4·221
14	1·761	2·145	2·624	2·977	3·787	4·140
15	1·753	2·131	2·602	2·947	3·733	4·073
16	1·746	2·120	2·583	2·921	3·686	4·015
17	1·740	2·110	2·567	2·898	3·646	3·965
18	1·734	2·101	2·552	2·878	3·610	3·922
19	1·729	2·093	2·539	2·861	3·579	3·883
20	1·725	2·086	2·528	2·845	3·552	3·850
21	1·721	2·080	2·518	2·831	3·527	3·819
22	1·717	2·074	2·508	2·819	3·505	3·792
23	1·714	2·069	2·500	2·807	3·485	3·767
24	1·711	2·064	2·492	2·797	3·467	3·745
25	1·708	2·060	2·485	2·787	3·450	3·725
26	1·706	2·056	2·479	2·779	3·435	3.707
27	1·703	2·052	2·473	2·771	3·421	3·690
28	1·701	2·048	2·467	2·763	3·408	3·674
29	1·699	2·045	2·462	2·756	3·396	3·659
30	1·697	2·042	2·457	2·750	3·385	3·646

Appendix 2. The χ^2 distribution.

The table gives the percentage points most frequently required for significance tests based on χ^2. Thus the probability of observing a χ^2 with 5 degrees of freedom *greater* in value than 11·07 is 0·05 or 5 per cent. Again, the probability of observing a χ^2 with 5 degrees of freedom *smaller* in value than 0·554 is $1 - 0·99 = 0·01$ or 1 per cent.

Degrees of freedom	Value of P				
	0·99	0·95	0·05	0·01	0·001
1	0·000157	0·00393	3·841	6·635	10·83
2	0·0201	0·103	5·991	9·210	13·82
3	0·115	0·352	7·815	11·34	16·27
4	0·297	0·711	9·488	13·28	18·47
5	0·554	1·145	11·07	15·09	20·51
6	0·872	1·635	12·59	16·81	22·46
7	1·239	2·167	14·07	18·48	24·32
8	1·646	2·733	15·51	20·09	26·13
9	2·088	3·325	16·92	21·67	27·88
10	2·558	3·940	18·31	23·21	29·59
11	3·053	4·575	19·68	24·72	31·26
12	3·571	5·226	21·03	26·22	32·91
13	4·107	5·892	22·36	27·69	34·53
14	4·660	6·571	23·68	29·14	36·12
15	5·229	7·261	25·00	30·58	37·70
16	5·812	7·962	26·30	32·00	39·25
17	6·408	8·672	27·59	33·41	40·79
18	7·015	9·390	28·87	34·81	42·31
19	7·633	10·12	30·14	36·19	43·82
20	8·260	10·85	31·41	37·57	45·31
21	8·897	11·59	32·67	38·93	46·80
22	9·542	12·34	33·92	40·29	48·27
23	10·20	13·09	35·17	41·64	49·73
24	10·86	13·85	36·42	42·98	51·18
25	11·52	14·61	37·65	44·31	52·62
26	12·20	15·38	38·89	45·64	54·05
27	12·88	16·15	40·11	46·96	55·48
28	13·56	16·93	41·34	48·28	56·89
29	14·26	17·71	42·56	49·59	58·30
30	14·95	18·49	43·77	50·89	59·70

Appendix 3. The correlation coefficient.
The table gives percentage points for the distribution of the estimated correlation coefficient r. Thus when there are 10 degrees of freedom (i.e. in samples of 12) the probability of observing an r greater in *absolute value* than 0·576 (i.e. < -0.576 or $> +0.576$) is 0·05 or 5 per cent.

Degrees of freedom	Values of P				
	0·10	0·05	0·02	0·01	0·001
1	0·9877	0·99692	0·99951	0·99988	0·9999988
2	0·9000	0·9500	0·9800	0·9900	0·9990
3	0·805	0·878	0·9343	0·9587	0·9911
4	0·729	0·811	0·882	0·9172	0·9741
5	0·669	0·754	0·833	0·875	0·9509
6	0·621	0·707	0·789	0·834	0·9249
7	0·582	0·666	0·750	0·798	0·898
8	0·549	0·632	0·715	0·765	0·872
9	0·521	0·602	0·685	0·735	0·847
10	0·497	0·576	0·658	0·708	0·823
11	0·476	0·553	0·634	0·684	0·801
12	0·457	0·532	0·612	0·661	0·780
13	0·441	0·514	0·592	0·641	0·760
14	0·426	0·497	0·574	0·623	0·742
15	0·412	0·482	0·558	0·606	0·725
16	0·400	0·468	0·543	0·590	0·708
17	0·389	0·456	0·529	0·575	0·693
18	0·378	0·444	0·516	0·561	0·679
19	0·369	0·433	0·503	0·549	0·665
20	0·360	0·423	0·492	0·537	0·652
25	0·323	0·381	0·445	0·487	0·597
30	0·296	0·349	0·409	0·449	0·554
35	0·275	0·325	0·381	0·418	0·519
40	0·257	0·304	0·358	0·393	0·490
45	0·243	0·288	0·338	0·372	0·465
50	0·231	0·273	0·322	0·354	0·443
60	0·211	0·250	0·295	0·325	0·408
70	0·195	0·232	0·274	0·302	0·380
80	0·183	0·217	0·257	0·283	0·357
90	0·173	0·205	0·242	0·267	0·338
100	0·164	0·195	0·230	0·254	0·321

Appendix 4. The z-transformation of correlation coefficient r.

r	z	r	z
0·00	0·0000	0·35	0·3654
0·01	0·0100	0·36	0·3769
0·02	0·0200	0·37	0·3884
0·03	0·0300	0·38	0·4001
0·04	0·0400	0·39	0·4118
0·05	0·0500	0·40	0·4236
0·06	0·0601	0·41	0·4356
0·07	0·0701	0·42	0·4477
0·08	0·0802	0·43	0·4599
0·09	0·0902	0·44	0·4722
0·10	0·1003	0·45	0·4847
0·11	0·1104	0·46	0·4973
0·12	0·1206	0·47	0·5101
0·13	0·1307	0·48	0·5230
0·14	0·1409	0·49	0·5361
0·15	0·1511	0·50	0·5493
0·16	0·1614	0·51	0·5627
0·17	0·1717	0·52	0·5763
0·18	0·1820	0·53	0·5901
0·19	0·1923	0·54	0·6042
0·20	0·2027	0·55	0·6184
0·21	0·2132	0·56	0·6328
0·22	0·2237	0·57	0·6475
0·23	0·2342	0·58	0·6625
0·24	0·2448	0·59	0·6777
0·25	0·2554	0·60	0·6931
0·26	0·2661	0·61	0·7089
0·27	0·2769	0·62	0·7250
0·28	0·2877	0·63	0·7414
0·29	0·2986	0·64	0·7582
0·30	0·3095	0·65	0·7753
0·31	0·3205	0·66	0·7928
0·32	0·3316	0·67	0·8107
0·33	0·3428	0·68	0·8291
0·34	0·3541	0·69	0·8480

Appendix 4—continued

r	z	r	z
0·70	0·8673	0·85	1·2562
0·71	0·8872	0·86	1·2933
0·72	0·9076	0·87	1·3331
0·73	0·9287	0·88	1·3758
0·74	0·9505	0·89	1·4219
0·75	0·9730	0·90	1·4722
0·76	0·9962	0·91	1·5275
0·77	1·0203	0·92	1·5890
0·78	1·0454	0·93	1·6584
0·79	1·0714	0·94	1·7380
0·80	1·0986	0·95	1·8318
0·81	1·1270	0·96	1·9459
0·82	1·1568	0·97	2·0923
0·83	1·1881	0·98	2·2976
0·84	1·2212	0·99	2·6467

Appendix 5. Table of *x* and *a* for values of *q* from $q = 0.01\%$ to $q = 30.0\%$. *q* is the incidence; *x* is the normal deviate (single-tailed) exceeded by the proportion *q*; *a* is the mean deviation of these individuals. Note changes of interval in *q* at $q = 2.0\%$ and $q = 21.0\%$.

q%	x	a	q%	x	a	q%	x	a	q%	x	a
0·01	3·719	3·960	0·40	2·652	2·962	0·80	2·409	2·740	1·20	2·257	2·603
0·02	3·540	3·790	0·41	2·644	2·954	0·81	2·404	2·736	1·21	2·254	2·600
0·03	3·432	3·687	0·42	2·636	2·947	0·82	2·400	2·732	1·22	2·251	2·597
0·04	3·353	3·613	0·43	2·628	2·939	0·83	2·395	2·728	1·23	2·248	2·594
0·05	3·291	3·554	0·44	2·620	2·932	0·84	2·391	2·724	1·24	2·244	2·591
0·06	3·239	3·507	0·45	2·612	2·925	0·85	2·387	2·720	1·25	2·241	2·589
0·07	3·195	3·464	0·46	2·605	2·918	0·86	2·382	2·716	1·26	2·238	2·586
0·08	3·156	3·429	0·47	2·597	2·911	0·87	2·378	2·712	1·27	2·235	2·583
0·09	3·121	3·397	0·48	2·590	2·905	0·88	2·374	2·708	1·28	2·232	2·580
0·10	3·090	3·367	0·49	2·583	2·898	0·89	2·370	2·704	1·29	2·229	2·578
0·11	3·062	3·341	0·50	2·576	2·892	0·90	2·366	2·701	1·30	2·226	2·575
0·12	3·036	3·317	0·51	2·569	2·886	0·91	2·361	2·697	1·31	2·223	2·572
0·13	3·012	3·294	0·52	2·562	2·880	0·92	2·357	2·693	1·32	2·220	2·570
0·14	2·989	3·273	0·53	2·556	2·873	0·93	2·353	2·690	1·33	2·217	2·567
0·15	2·968	3·253	0·54	2·549	2·868	0·94	2·349	2·686	1·34	2·214	2·564
0·16	2·948	3·234	0·55	2·543	2·862	0·95	2·346	2·683	1·35	2·211	2·562
0·17	2·929	3·217	0·56	2·536	2·856	0·96	2·342	2·679	1·36	2·209	2·559
0·18	2·911	3·201	0·57	2·530	2·850	0·97	2·338	2·676	1·37	2·206	2·557
0·19	2·894	3·185	0·58	2·524	2·845	0·98	2·334	2·672	1·38	2·203	2·554
			0·59	2·518	2·839	0·99	2·330	2·669	1·39	2·200	2·552

Appendix 5—continued

q%	x	a	q%	x	a	q%	a	a	q%	x	a
0·20	2·878	3·170	0·60	2·512	2·834	1·00	2·326	2·665	1·40	2·197	2·549
0·21	2·863	3·156	0·61	2·506	2·829	1·01	2·323	2·662	1·41	2·194	2·547
0·22	2·848	3·142	0·62	2·501	2·823	1·02	2·319	2·658	1·42	2·192	2·544
0·23	2·834	3·129	0·63	2·495	2·818	1·03	2·315	2·655	1·43	2·189	2·542
0·24	2·820	3·117	0·64	2·489	2·813	1·04	2·312	2·652	1·44	2·186	2·539
0·25	2·807	3·104	0·65	2·484	2·808	1·05	2·308	2·649	1·45	2·183	2·537
0·26	2·794	3·093	0·66	2·478	2·803	1·06	2·304	2·645	1·46	2·181	2·534
0·27	2·782	3·081	0·67	2·473	2·798	1·07	2·301	2·642	1·47	2·178	2·532
0·28	2·770	3·070	0·68	2·468	2·793	1·08	2·297	2·639	1·48	2·175	2·529
0·29	2·759	3·060	0·69	2·462	2·789	1·09	2·294	2·636	1·49	2·173	2·527
0·30	2·748	3·050	0·70	2·457	2·784	1·10	2·290	2·633	1·50	2·170	2·525
0·31	2·737	3·040	0·71	2·452	2·779	1·11	2·287	2·630	1·51	2·167	2·522
0·32	2·727	3·030	0·72	2·447	2·775	1·12	2·283	2·627	1·52	2·165	2·520
0·33	2·716	3·021	0·73	2·442	2·770	1·13	2·280	2·624	1·53	2·162	2·518
0·34	2·706	3·012	0·74	2·437	2·766	1·14	2·277	2·621	1·54	2·160	2·515
0·35	2·697	3·003	0·75	2·432	2·761	1·15	2·273	2·618	1·55	2·157	2·513
0·36	2·687	2·994	0·76	2·428	2·757	1·16	2·270	2·615	1·56	2·155	2·511
0·37	2·678	2·986	0·77	2·423	2·753	1·17	2·267	2·612	1·57	2·152	2·508
0·38	2·669	2·978	0·78	2·418	2·748	1·18	2·264	2·609	1·58	2·149	2·506
0·39	2·661	2·969	0·79	2·414	2·744	1·19	2·260	2·606	1·59	2·147	2·504

Appendix 5—continued

q%	x	a	q%	x	a	q%	x	a	q%	x	a
1·60	2·144	2·502	2·0	2·054	2·421	6·0	1·555	1·985	10·0	1·282	1·755
1·61	2·142	2·499	2·1	2·034	2·403	6·1	1·546	1·978	10·1	1·276	1·750
1·62	2·139	2·497	2·2	2·014	2·386	6·2	1·538	1·971	10·2	1·270	1·746
1·63	2·137	2·495	2·3	1·995	2·369	6·3	1·530	1·964	10·3	1·265	1·741
1·64	2·135	2·493	2·4	1·977	2·353	6·4	1·522	1·957	10·4	1·259	1·736
1·65	2·132	2·491	2·5	1·960	2·338	6·5	1·514	1·951	10·5	1·254	1·732
1·66	2·130	2·489	2·6	1·943	2·323	6·6	1·506	1·944	10·6	1·248	1·727
1·67	2·127	2·486	2·7	1·927	2·309	6·7	1·499	1·937	10·7	1·243	1·723
1·68	2·125	2·484	2·8	1·911	2·295	6·8	1·491	1·931	10·8	1·237	1·718
1·69	2·122	2·482	2·9	1·896	2·281	6·9	1·483	1·924	10·9	1·232	1·714
1·70	2·120	2·480	3·0	1·881	2·268	7·0	1·476	1·918	11·0	1·227	1·709
1·71	2·118	2·478	3·1	1·866	2·255	7·1	1·468	1·912	11·1	1·221	1·705
1·72	2·115	2·476	3·2	1·852	2·243	7·2	1·461	1·906	11·2	1·216	1·701
1·73	2·113	2·474	3·3	1·838	2·231	7·3	1·454	1·899	11·3	1·211	1·696
1·74	2·111	2·472	3·4	1·825	2·219	7·4	1·447	1·893	11·4	1·206	1·692
1·75	2·108	2·470	3·5	1·812	2·208	7·5	1·440	1·887	11·5	1·200	1·688
1·76	2·106	2·467	3·6	1·799	2·197	7·6	1·433	1·881	11·6	1·195	1·684
1·77	2·104	2·465	3·7	1·787	2·186	7·7	1·426	1·876	11·7	1·190	1·679
1·78	2·101	2·463	3·8	1·774	2·175	7·8	1·419	1·870	11·8	1·185	1·675
1·79	2·099	2·461	3·9	1·762	2·165	7·9	1·412	1·864	11·9	1·180	1·671

Appendix 5—continued

q%	x	a	q%	x	a	q%	x	a	q%	x	a
1·80	2·097	2·459	4·0	1·751	2·154	8·0	1·405	1·858	12·0	1·175	1·667
1·81	2·095	2·457	4·1	1·739	2·144	8·1	1·398	1·853	12·1	1·170	1·663
1·82	2·092	2·455	4·2	1·728	2·135	8·2	1·392	1·847	12·2	1·165	1·659
1·83	2·090	2·453	4·3	1·717	2·125	8·3	1·385	1·842	12·3	1·160	1·655
1·84	2·088	2·451	4·4	1·706	2·116	8·4	1·379	1·836	12·4	1·155	1·651
1·85	2·086	2·449	4·5	1·695	2·106	8·5	1·372	1·831	12·5	1·150	1·647
1·86	2·084	2·447	4·6	1·685	2·097	8·6	1·366	1·825	12·6	1·146	1·643
1·87	2·081	2·445	4·7	1·675	2·088	8·7	1·359	1·820	12·7	1·141	1·639
1·88	2·079	2·444	4·8	1·665	2·080	8·8	1·353	1·815	12·8	1·136	1·635
1·89	2·077	2·442	4·9	1·655	2·071	8·9	1·347	1·810	12·9	1·131	1·631
1·90	2·075	2·440	5·0	1·645	2·063	9·0	1·341	1·804	13·0	1·126	1·627
1·91	2·073	2·438	5·1	1·635	2·054	9·1	1·335	1·799	13·1	1·122	1·623
1·92	2·071	2·436	5·2	1·626	2·046	9·2	1·329	1·794	13·2	1·117	1·620
1·93	2·068	2·434	5·3	1·616	2·038	9·3	1·323	1·789	13·3	1·112	1·616
1·94	2·066	2·432	5·4	1·607	2·030	9·4	1·317	1·784	13·4	1·108	1·612
1·95	2·064	2·430	5·5	1·598	2·023	9·5	1·311	1·779	13·5	1·103	1·608
1·96	2·062	2·428	5·6	1·589	2·015	9·6	1·305	1·774	13·6	1·098	1·605
1·97	2·060	2·426	5·7	1·580	2·007	9·7	1·299	1·769	13·7	1·094	1·601
1·98	2·058	2·425	5·8	1·572	2·000	9·8	1·293	1·765	13·8	1·089	1·597
1·99	2·056	2·423	5·9	1·563	1·993	9·9	1·287	1·760	13·9	1·085	1·593

Appendix 5—continued

q%	x	a	q%	x	a	q%	x	a	q%	x	a
14·0	1·080	1·590	16·0	0·994	1·521	18·0	0·915	1·458	20·0	0·842	1·400
14·1	1·076	1·586	16·1	0·990	1·517	18·1	0·912	1·455	20·1	0·838	1·397
14·2	1·071	1·583	16·2	0·986	1·514	18·2	0·908	1·452	20·2	0·834	1·394
14·3	1·067	1·579	16·3	0·982	1·511	18·3	0·904	1·449	20·3	0·831	1·391
14·4	1·063	1·575	16·4	0·978	1·508	18·4	0·900	1·446	20·4	0·827	1·389
14·5	1·058	1·572	16·5	0·974	1·504	18·5	0·896	1·443	20·5	0·824	1·386
14·6	1·054	1·568	16·6	0·970	1·501	18·6	0·893	1·440	20·6	0·820	1·383
14·7	1·049	1·565	16·7	0·966	1·498	18·7	0·889	1·437	20·7	0·817	1·381
14·8	1·045	1·561	16·8	0·962	1·495	18·8	0·885	1·434	20·8	0·813	1·378
14·9	1·041	1·558	16·9	0·958	1·492	18·9	0·882	1·431	20·9	0·810	1·375
15·0	1·036	1·554	17·0	0·954	1·489	19·0	0·878	1·428	21·0	0·806	1·372
15·1	1·032	1·551	17·1	0·950	1·485	19·1	0·874	1·425	22·0	0·772	1·346
15·2	1·028	1·548	17·2	0·946	1·482	19·2	0·871	1·422	23·0	0·739	1·320
15·3	1·024	1·544	17·3	0·942	1·479	19·3	0·867	1·420	24·0	0·706	1·295
15·4	1·019	1·541	17·4	0·938	1·476	19·4	0·863	1·417			
15·5	1·015	1·537	17·5	0·935	1·473	19·5	0·860	1·414	25·0	0·674	1·271
15·6	1·011	1·534	17·6	0·931	1·470	19·6	0·856	1·411	26·0	0·643	1·248
15·7	1·007	1·531	17·7	0·927	1·467	19·7	0·852	1·408	27·0	0·613	1·225
15·8	1·003	1·527	17·8	0·923	1·464	19·8	0·849	1·405	28·0	0·583	1·202
15·9	0·999	1·524	17·9	0·919	1·461	19·9	0·845	1·403	29·0	0·553	1·180
									30·0	0·524	1·159

Appendix 6. Linkage (lod) scores for families with up to seven children.

No.	Scored children count		0·01	0·05	0·1	0·15	0·2	0·25	0·3	0·35	0·4	0·45
							Recombination fraction (θ)					
1.	1 n−r	0 r	0·297	0·279	0·255	0·230	0·204	0·176	0·146	0·114	0·079	0·041
	0 n−r	1 r	−1·699	−1·000	−0·699	−0·523	−0·398	−0·301	−0·222	−0·155	−0·097	−0·046
2.	2 n−r	0 r	0·593	0·558	0·511	0·461	0·408	0·352	0·292	0·228	0·158	0·083
	1 n−r	1 r	−1·402	−0·721	−0·444	−0·292	−0·194	−0·125	−0·076	−0·041	−0·018	−0·004
	0 n−r	2 r	−3·398	−2·000	−1·398	−1·046	−0·796	−0·602	−0·444	−0·310	−0·194	−0·092
	z_1 2:0		0·292	0·258	0·215	0·173	0·134	0·097	0·064	0·037	0·017	0·004
	z_1 2:0	e_1 2:0	0·460	0·395	0·319	0·250	0·190	0·135	0·088	0·050	0·023	0·005
	z_1 2:0	e_1 1:1	0·171	0·154	0·131	0·107	0·085	0·062	0·041	0·024	0·011	0·003
	z_1 1:1		−1·402	−0·721	−0·444	−0·292	−0·194	−0·125	−0·076	−0·041	−0·018	−0·004
	z_1 1:1	e_1 2:0	−1·234	−0·584	−0·340	−0·215	−0·138	−0·087	−0·052	−0·028	−0·012	−0·003
	z_1 1:1	e_1 1:1	−1·523	−0·825	−0·528	−0·358	−0·243	−0·160	−0·099	−0·054	−0·024	−0·006
3.	3 n−r	0 r	0·890	0·836	0·766	0·691	0·612	0·528	0·438	0·342	0·238	0·124
	2 n−r	1 r	−1·106	−0·442	−0·188	−0·062	0·010	0·051	0·070	0·073	0·061	0·037
	1 n−r	2 r	−3·101	−1·721	−1·143	−0·815	−0·592	−0·426	−0·298	−0·196	−0·115	−0·050
	0 n−r	3 r	−5·097	−3·000	−2·097	−1·569	−1·194	−0·903	−0·666	−0·465	−0·291	−0·137
	z_1 3:0		0·589	0·535	0·465	0·393	0·318	0·243	0·170	0·104	0·049	0·013
	z_1 3:0	e_1 3:0	0·819	0·720	0·605	0·495	0·391	0·292	0·201	0·121	0·057	0·015
	z_1 3:0	e_1 2:1	0·533	0·487	0·427	0·364	0·296	0·228	0·160	0·098	0·047	0·013
	z_1 2:1		−1·402	−0·721	−0·444	−0·292	−0·194	−0·125	−0·076	−0·041	−0·018	−0·004
	z_1 2:1	e_1 3:0	−1·172	−0·536	−0·305	−0·190	−0·121	−0·076	−0·045	−0·024	−0·010	−0·002
	z_1 2:1	e_1 2:1	−1·458	−0·769	−0·482	−0·321	−0·216	−0·140	−0·086	−0·047	−0·020	−0·004

Appendix 6—continued

No.	Scored children	count	0·01	0·05	0·1	0·15	0·2	0·25	0·3	0·35	0·4	0·45
			Recombination fraction (θ)									
4.	4 $n-r$	0 r	1·187	1·115	1·021	0·922	0·816	0·704	0·585	0·456	0·317	0·166
	3 $n-r$	1 r	−0·809	−0·164	0·067	0·168	0·214	0·227	0·217	0·187	0·141	0·078
	2 $n-r$	2 r	−2·805	−1·442	−0·887	−0·585	−0·388	−0·250	−0·151	−0·082	−0·035	−0·009
	1 $n-r$	3 r	−4·800	−2·721	−1·842	−1·338	−0·990	−0·727	−0·519	−0·351	−0·212	−0·096
	0 $n-r$	4 r	−6·796	−4·000	−2·796	−2·092	−1·592	−1·204	−0·887	−0·620	−0·388	−0·183
	z_1 4:0		0·886	0·814	0·720	0·621	0·517	0·409	0·298	0·190	0·094	0·025
	z_1 4:0	e_1 4:0	1·142	1·013	0·865	0·724	0·589	0·457	0·328	0·206	0·101	0·027
	z_1 4:0	e_1 3:1	0·860	0·795	0·708	0·614	0·513	0·407	0·298	0·190	0·094	0·025
	z_1 4:0	e_1 2:2	0·858	0·787	0·696	0·600	0·500	0·397	0·290	0·185	0·092	0·025
	z_1 3:1		−1·110	−0·464	−0·229	−0·119	−0·060	−0·028	−0·011	−0·004	0·000	0·000
	z_1 3:1	e_1 4:0	−0·854	−0·265	−0·084	−0·016	0·012	0·020	0·019	0·012	0·007	0·002
	z_1 3:1	e_1 3:1	−1·136	−0·483	−0·241	−0·126	−0·064	−0·030	−0·011	−0·004	0·000	0·000
	z_1 3:1	e_1 2:2	−1·138	−0·491	−0·253	−0·140	−0·077	−0·040	−0·019	−0·009	−0·002	0·000
	z_1 2:2		−2·805	−1·442	−0·887	−0·585	−0·388	−0·250	−0·151	−0·082	−0·035	−0·009
	z_1 2:2	e_1 4:0	−2·549	−1·243	−0·742	−0·482	−0·316	−0·202	−0·121	−0·066	−0·028	−0·007
	z_1 2:2	e_1 3:1	−2·831	−1·461	−0·899	−0·592	−0·392	−0·252	−0·151	−0·082	−0·035	−0·009
	z_1 2:2	e_1 2:2	−2·833	−1·469	−0·911	−0·606	−0·405	−0·262	−0·159	−0·087	−0·037	−0·009
5.	5 $n-r$	0 r	1·483	1·394	1·276	1·152	1·021	0·880	0·731	0·570	0·396	0·207
	4 $n-r$	1 r	−0·512	0·115	0·322	0·399	0·419	0·403	0·363	0·301	0·220	0·120
	3 $n-r$	2 r	−2·508	−1·164	−0·632	−0·354	−0·184	−0·074	−0·005	−0·032	0·044	0·033
	2 $n-r$	3 r	−4·504	−2·442	−1·586	−1·108	−0·786	−0·551	−0·373	−0·237	−0·132	−0·054
	1 $n-r$	4 r	−6·499	−3·721	−2·541	−1·861	−1·388	−1·028	−0·741	−0·506	−0·308	−0·142
	0 $n-r$	5 r	−8·495	−5·000	−3·495	−2·614	−1·990	−1·505	−1·109	−0·775	−0·485	−0·229
	z_1 5:0		1·182	1·093	0·975	0·851	0·720	0·581	0·436	0·288	0·149	0·042
	z_1 5:0	e_1 5:0	1·448	1·292	1·113	0·946	0·784	0·622	0·461	0·301	0·155	0·043

No.	Scored children count		Recombination fraction (θ)									
			0·01	0·05	0·1	0·15	0·2	0·25	0·3	0·35	0·4	0·45
	z_1 5:0	e_1 4:1	1·170	1·088	0·975	0·855	0·725	0·585	0·439	0·290	0·150	0·042
	z_1 5:0	e_1 3:2	1·168	1·080	0·963	0·841	0·712	0·575	0·432	0·286	0·148	0·042
	z_1 4:1		−0·813	−0·186	0·022	0·100	0·124	0·118	0·095	0·063	0·031	0·008
	z_1 4:1	e_1 5:0	−0·547	−0·013	0·160	0·195	0·182	0·159	0·120	0·076	0·037	0·009
	z_1 4:1	e_1 4:1	−0·825	−0·191	0·022	0·104	0·129	0·122	0·098	0·065	0·032	0·008
	z_1 4:1	e_1 3:2	−0·827	−0·199	0·010	0·090	0·116	0·112	0·091	0·061	0·030	0·008
	z_1 3:2		−2·805	−1·442	−0·887	−0·585	−0·388	−0·250	−0·151	−0·082	−0·035	−0·009
	z_1 3:2	e_1 5:0	−2·539	−1·243	−0·749	−0·490	−0·324	−0·209	−0·126	−0·069	−0·029	−0·008
	z_1 3:2	e_1 4:1	−2·817	−1·447	−0·887	−0·581	−0·383	−0·246	−0·148	−0·080	−0·034	−0·009
	z_1 3:2	e_1 3:2	−2·819	−1·455	−0·899	−0·595	−0·396	−0·256	−0·155	−0·084	−0·036	−0·009
6.	6 $n-r$	0 r	1·780	1·673	1·532	1·383	1·225	1·057	0·877	0·684	0·475	0·248
	5 $n-r$	1 r	−0·216	0·394	0·577	0·629	0·623	0·579	0·509	0·415	0·299	0·161
	4 $n-r$	2 r	−2·211	−0·885	−0·377	−0·124	0·021	0·102	0·141	0·146	0·123	0·074
	3 $n-r$	3 r	−4·207	−2·164	−1·331	−0·877	−0·581	−0·375	−0·227	−0·123	−0·053	−0·013
	2 $n-r$	4 r	−6·203	−3·442	−2·285	−1·631	−1·184	−0·852	−0·595	−0·392	−0·229	−0·100
	1 $n-r$	5 r	−8·198	−4·721	−3·240	−2·384	−1·786	−1·329	−0·963	−0·661	−0·405	−0·187
	0 $n-r$	6 r	−10·194	−6·000	−4·194	−3·137	−2·388	−1·806	−1·331	−0·929	−0·581	−0·275
	z_1 6:0	e_1 6:0	1·479	1·371	1·231	1·082	0·924	0·756	0·578	0·393	0·211	0·061
	z_1 6:0	e_1 5:1	1·748	1·563	1·358	1·166	0·978	0·790	0·598	0·403	0·215	0·062
	z_1 6:0	e_1 4:2	1·474	1·373	1·237	1·090	0·932	0·762	0·583	0·396	0·212	0·061
	z_1 6:0	e_1 3:3	1·472	1·365	1·226	1·078	0·921	0·754	0·577	0·393	0·211	0·061
	z_1 6:0		1·472	1·364	1·224	1·076	0·919	0·752	0·575	0·391	0·211	0·061
	z_1 5:1	e_1 6:0	−0·517	0·093	0·276	0·329	0·323	0·284	0·222	0·149	0·076	0·021
	z_1 5:1	e_1 5:1	−0·248	0·285	0·403	0·413	0·377	0·318	0·242	0·159	0·080	0·022
	z_1 5:1	e_1 4:2	−0·522	0·095	0·283	0·337	0·331	0·290	0·227	0·152	0·077	0·021
	z_1 5:1	e_1 3:3	−0·524	0·087	0·271	0·325	0·320	0·282	0·221	0·149	0·076	0·021
	z_1 5:1		−0·524	0·086	0·269	0·323	0·318	0·280	0·219	0·147	0·076	0·021
	z_1 4:2		−2·512	−1·185	−0·673	−0·412	−0·254	−0·153	−0·087	−0·044	−0·018	−0·004

Appendix 6—continued

No.	Scored children count		Recombination fraction (θ)									
			0·01	0·05	0·1	0·15	0·2	0·25	0·3	0·35	0·4	0·45
	z_1 4:2	e_1 6:0	−2·243	−0·993	−0·546	−0·328	−0·200	−0·119	−0·067	−0·034	−0·014	−0·003
	z_1 4:2	e_1 5:1	−2·517	−1·183	−0·667	−0·404	−0·246	−0·147	−0·082	−0·041	−0·017	−0·004
	z_1 4:2	e_1 4:2	−2·519	−1·191	−0·678	−0·416	−0·257	−0·155	−0·088	−0·044	−0·018	−0·004
	z_1 4:2	e_1 3:3	−2·519	−1·192	−0·680	−0·418	−0·259	−0·157	−0·090	−0·046	−0·018	−0·004
	z_1 3:3	e_1 6:0	−4·207	−2·164	−1·331	−0·877	−0·581	−0·375	−0·227	−0·123	−0·053	−0·013
	z_1 3:3	e_1 5:1	−3·938	−1·972	−1·204	−0·793	−0·527	−0·341	−0·207	−0·113	−0·049	−0·012
	z_1 3:3	e_1 4:2	−4·212	−2·162	−1·325	−0·869	−0·573	−0·369	−0·222	−0·120	−0·052	−0·013
	z_1 3:3	e_1 4:2	−4·214	−2·170	−1·336	−0·881	−0·584	−0·377	−0·228	−0·123	−0·053	−0·013
	z_1 3:3	e_1 3:3	−4·214	−2·171	−1·338	−0·883	−0·586	−0·397	−0·230	−0·125	−0·053	−0·013
7.	7 $n-r$	0 r	2·077	1·951	1·787	1·613	1·429	1·233	1·023	0·798	0·554	0·290
	6 $n-r$	1 r	0·081	0·673	0·833	0·860	0·827	0·756	0·655	0·529	0·378	0·203
	5 $n-r$	2 r	−1·915	−0·606	−0·122	0·106	0·225	0·278	0·287	0·260	0·202	0·115
	4 $n-r$	3 r	−3·910	−1·885	−1·076	−0·647	−0·377	−0·199	−0·081	−0·009	0·026	0·028
	3 $n-r$	4 r	−5·906	−3·164	−2·030	−1·400	−0·979	−0·676	−0·449	−0·278	−0·150	−0·059
	2 $n-r$	5 r	−7·902	−4·442	−2·984	−2·153	−1·581	−1·153	−0·817	−0·547	−0·326	−0·146
	1 $n-r$	6 r	−9·897	−5·721	−3·939	−2·907	−2·184	−1·630	−1·185	−0·815	−0·502	−0·233
	0 $n-r$	7 r	−11·893	−7·000	−4·893	−3·660	−2·787	−2·107	−1·553	−1·084	−0·678	−0·320
	z_1 7:0	e_1 7:0	1·776	1·650	1·486	1·312	1·128	0·932	0·723	0·502	0·278	0·084
	z_1 7:0	e_1 6:1	2·045	1·833	1·601	1·384	1·173	0·959	0·738	0·510	0·281	0·084
	z_1 7:0	e_1 5:2	1·775	1·655	1·494	1·321	1·136	0·938	0·727	0·505	0·279	0·084
	z_1 7:0	e_1 4:3	1·773	1·647	1·484	1·311	1·128	0·932	0·723	0·502	0·278	0·084
	z_1 7:0		1·773	1·647	1·483	1·309	1·125	0·930	0·722	0·502	0·278	0·084
	z_1 6:1	e_1 7:0	−0·220	0·371	0·532	0·559	0·526	0·456	0·360	0·247	0·131	0·037
	z_1 6:1	e_1 6:1	0·049	0·554	0·647	0·631	0·571	0·483	0·375	0·255	0·134	0·037
	z_1 6:1	e_1 5:2	−0·221	0·376	0·540	0·568	0·534	0·462	0·364	0·250	0·132	0·037
	z_1 6:1		−0·223	0·368	0·530	0·558	0·526	0·456	0·360	0·247	0·131	0·037

Appendix 6—continued

No.	Scored children count	0·01	0·05	0·1	0·15	Recombination fraction (θ) 0·2	0·25	0·3	0·35	0·4	0·45
z_1 6:1	e_1 4:3	$-0\cdot223$	$0\cdot368$	$0\cdot529$	$0\cdot556$	$0\cdot523$	$0\cdot454$	$0\cdot359$	$0\cdot247$	$0\cdot131$	$0\cdot037$
z_1 5:2		$-2\cdot216$	$-0\cdot907$	$-0\cdot422$	$-0\cdot192$	$-0\cdot070$	$-0\cdot007$	$0\cdot019$	$0\cdot022$	$0\cdot014$	$0\cdot004$
z_1 5:2	e_1 7:0	$-1\cdot947$	$-0\cdot724$	$-0\cdot307$	$-0\cdot120$	$-0\cdot025$	$0\cdot020$	$0\cdot034$	$0\cdot030$	$0\cdot017$	$0\cdot004$
z_1 5:2	e_1 6:1	$-2\cdot217$	$-0\cdot902$	$-0\cdot414$	$-0\cdot183$	$-0\cdot062$	$-0\cdot001$	$0\cdot023$	$0\cdot025$	$0\cdot015$	$0\cdot004$
z_1 5:2	e_1 5:2	$-2\cdot219$	$-0\cdot910$	$-0\cdot424$	$-0\cdot193$	$-0\cdot071$	$-0\cdot007$	$0\cdot019$	$0\cdot022$	$0\cdot014$	$0\cdot004$
z_1 5:2	e_1 4:3	$-2\cdot219$	$-0\cdot910$	$-0\cdot425$	$-0\cdot195$	$-0\cdot073$	$-0\cdot009$	$0\cdot018$	$0\cdot022$	$0\cdot014$	$0\cdot004$
z_1 4:3		$-4\cdot207$	$-2\cdot164$	$-1\cdot331$	$-0\cdot877$	$-0\cdot581$	$-0\cdot375$	$-0\cdot227$	$-0\cdot123$	$-0\cdot053$	$-0\cdot013$
z_1 4:3	e_1 7:0	$-3\cdot938$	$-1\cdot981$	$-1\cdot216$	$-0\cdot805$	$-0\cdot536$	$-0\cdot348$	$-0\cdot212$	$-0\cdot115$	$-0\cdot050$	$-0\cdot013$
z_1 4:3	e_1 6:1	$-4\cdot208$	$-2\cdot159$	$-1\cdot323$	$-0\cdot868$	$-0\cdot573$	$-0\cdot369$	$-0\cdot223$	$-0\cdot120$	$-0\cdot052$	$-0\cdot013$
z_1 4:3	e_1 5:2	$-4\cdot210$	$-2\cdot167$	$-1\cdot353$	$-0\cdot878$	$-0\cdot581$	$-0\cdot375$	$-0\cdot227$	$-0\cdot123$	$-0\cdot053$	$-0\cdot013$
z_1 4:3	e_1 4:3	$-4\cdot210$	$-2\cdot167$	$-1\cdot334$	$-0\cdot880$	$-0\cdot584$	$-0\cdot377$	$-0\cdot228$	$-0\cdot124$	$-0\cdot053$	$-0\cdot013$

References

Aird, I. M., Bentall, H. H. & Roberts, J. A. F. (1953) A relationship between cancer of stomach and the ABO blood groups. *Brit. med. J., i,* 799–801.

Allen, G., Harvald, B. & Shields, J. (1967) Measures of twin concordance. *Acta. Genet. (Basel),* **17,** 475–81.

Allison, A. C. (1964) Polymorphism and natural selection in human populations. *Cold Spring Harbor Sympos. Quant. Biol.,* **29,** 137–49.

Armitage, P. (1955). Tests for linear trends in proportions and frequencies. *Biometrics,* **11,** 375–86.

Armitage, P. (1971) *Statistical Methods in Medical Research.* Oxford: Blackwell.

Ashley, D. J. B. & Davies, H. D. (1966) The use of the surname as a genetic marker in Wales. *J. Med. Genet.,* **3,** 203–11.

Bailey, N. T. J. (1951) The estimation of the frequencies of recessives with incomplete multiple selection. *Ann. Eugen. (Lond.),* **16,** 215–22.

Bajema, C. J. (Ed.) (1971) *Natural Selection in Human Populations.* New York: John Wiley.

Barton, D. E. & David, F. N. (1958) A test for birth order effect. *Ann. Hum. Genet. (Lond.),* **22,** 250–7.

Bayes, T. (1763) An essay towards solving a problem in the doctrine of chances. *Philos. Trans.,* **53,** 376–418.

Benirschke, K. & Kim, C. K. (1973) Multiple pregnancy. *New Engl. J. Med.,* **288,** 1276–84 and 1329–36.

Blank, C. E. (1960) Apert's syndrome (a type of acrocephalosyndactyly)—observations on a British series of thirty-nine cases. *Ann. Hum. Genet. (Lond.),* **24,** 151–64.

Bodmer, W., Bodmer, J., Ihde, D. & Adler, S. (1969) Genetic and serological association analysis of the HL-A leukocyte system. In *Computer Applications in Genetics,* ed. Morton, N. E. 117–27. Honolulu: University of Hawaii Press.

Bonaiti-Pellié, C. & Smith, C. (1974) Risk tables for genetic counselling in some common congenital malformations. *J. Med. Genet.,* **11,** 374–7.

Brewerton, D. A., Caffrey, M., Hart, F. D., James, D. C. O., Nicholls, A. & Sturrock, R. D. (1973) Ankylosing spondylitis and HLA 27. *Lancet, i,* 904–7.

Bulmer, M. G. (1959) The effect of parental age, parity and duration of marriage on the twinning rate. *Ann. Hum. Genet. (Lond.),* **23,** 454–8.

Bulmer, M. G. (1970) *The Biology of Twinning in Man.* Oxford: Clarendon Press.

Bundey, S., Harrison, M. J. G. & Marsden, C. D. (1975) A genetic study of torsion dystonia. *J. Med. Genet.,* **12,** 12–9.

Burt, C. & Howard, M. (1956) The multifactorial theory of inheritance and its application to intelligence. *Brit. J. Statist. Psychol.,* **9(2),** 95–131.

Candela, P. B. (1942) The introduction of blood group B into Europe. *Hum. Biol.,* **14,** 413–43.

Carter, C. O. (1965) The inheritance of common congenital malformations. *Prog. Med. Genet.,* **4,** 59–84.

Carter, C. O. (1976) Genetics of common single malformations. *Brit. Med. Bull.,* **32,** 21–26.

Cavalli-Sforza, L. L. & Bodmer, W. F. (1971) *The Genetics of Human Populations.* San Francisco: Freeman.

Charlesworth, B. & Charlesworth, D. (1973) The measurement of fitness and mutation rate in human populations. *Ann. Hum. Genet. (Lond.),* **37,** 175–87.

Chen, S., Thompson, M. W. & Rose, V. (1971) Endocardial fibroelastosis: family studies with special reference to counseling. *J. Pediat.,* **79,** 385–92.

Clarke, C. A. (1959a) Distribution of ABO blood groups and the secretor status in duodenal ulcer families. *Gastroenterologia,* **92,** 99–103.

Clarke, C. A. (1959b). The relative fitness of human mutant genotypes. In *Natural Selection in Human Populations.* ed. Roberts, D. F. & Harrison, G. A. 17–34. London: Pergamon Press.

Clarke, C. A. (1961) Blood groups and disease. *Prog. Med. Genet.,* **1,** 81–119.

Conneally, P. M. & Heuch, I. (1974) A computer program to determine genetic risks—a simplified version of PEDIG. *Amer. J. Hum. Genet.,* **26,** 773–5.

Cross, H. E. & McKusick, V. A. (1967) The Mast syndrome. A recessively inherited form of presenile dementia with motor disturbances. *Arch. Neurol.,* **16,** 1–13.

Crow, J. F. & Mange, A. P. (1965) Measurement of inbreeding from the frequency of marriages between persons of the same surname. *Eugen. Quart.,* **12(4),** 199–203.

Curnow, R. N. (1972) The multifactorial model for the inheritance of liability to disease and its implications for relatives at risk. *Biometrics,* **28,** 931–46.

Dahlberg, G. (1947) *Mathematical Methods for Population Genetics.* Basle: Karger.

Danks, D. M., Allan, J. & Anderson, C. M. (1965) A genetic study of fibrocystic disease of the pancreas. *Ann. Hum. Genet. (Lond.),* **28,** 323–40.

Edwards, J. H. (1960) The simulation of Mendelism. *Acta Genet.,* **10,** 63–70.

Edwards, J. H. (1961) The recognition and estimation of cyclic trends. *Ann. Hum. Genet. (Lond.),* **25,** 83–7.

Edwards, J. H. (1965) The meaning of the associations between blood groups and disease. *Ann. Hum. Genet. (Lond.),* **29,** 77–83.

Edwards, J. H. (1968) The value of twins in genetic studies. *Proc. Royal Soc. Med.,* **61,** 227–9.

Edwards, J. H. (1969) Familial predisposition in man. *Brit. Med. Bull.,* **25,** 58–64.

Edwards, J. H. (1971) The analysis of X-linkage. *Ann. Hum. Genet. (Lond.),* **34,** 229–50.

Emery, A. E. H. (1965) Carrier detection in sex-linked muscular dystrophy. *J. Génèt. Hum.,* **14,** 318–29.

Emery, A. E. H. (1966) Genetic linkage between the loci for colour blindness and Duchenne type muscular dystrophy. *J. Med. Genet.,* **3,** 92–5.

Emery, A. E. H. (1975) *Elements of Medical Genetics,* 4th edition. Edinburgh: Churchill Livingstone.

Emery, A. E. H. & Lawrence, J. S. (1967) Genetics of ankylosing spondylitis. *J. Med. Genet.,* **4,** 239–44.

Emery, A. E. H. & Morton, R. (1968) Genetic counselling in lethal X-linked disorders. *Acta Genet. (Basel),* **18,** 534–42.

Emery, A. E. H., Smith, C. A. B. & Sanger, R. (1969) The linkage relations of the loci for benign (Becker type) X-borne muscular dystrophy, colour blindness and the Xg blood groups. *Ann. Hum. Genet. (Lond.),* **32,** 261–9.

Evans, D. A. P., Manley, K. A. & McKusick, V. A. (1960) Genetic control of isoniazid metabolism in man. *Brit. med. J.,* **2,** 485–91.

Falconer, D. S. (1960) *Introduction to Quantitative Genetics.* Edinburgh: Oliver and Boyd.

Falconer, D. S. (1965) The inheritance of liability to certain diseases estimated from the incidence among relatives. *Ann. Hum. Genet. (Lond.),* **29,** 51–76.

Falconer, D. S. (1967) The inheritance of liability to diseases with variable age of onset with particular reference to diabetes mellitus. *Ann. Hum. Genet. (Lond.),* **31,** 1–20.

Fedrick, J. (1970) Anencephalus: variation with maternal age, parity, social class and region in England, Scotland and Wales. *Ann. Hum. Genet. (Lond.),* **34,** 31–8.

Feltkamp, T. E. W., Van den Berg-Loonen, P. M., Nijenhuis, L. E., Engelfriet, C. P., Van Rossum, A. L., Van Loghem, J. J. & Oosterhuis, H. J. G. H. (1974) Myasthenia gravis, autoantibodies and HL-A antigens. *Brit. med. J., i,* 131–3.

Fisher, R. A. (1930) *The Genetical Theory of Natural Selection.* Oxford: Clarendon Press. Also available now as a paperback edition. (1958) New York: Dover Publications.

Fisher, R. A. (1934) The effect of methods of ascertainment upon the estimation of frequencies. *Ann. Eugen. (Lond.),* **6,** 13–25.

Fisher, R. A. (1970) *Statistical Methods for Research Workers,* 14th edition. Edinburgh: Oliver and Boyd.

Fisher, R. A. & Yates, F. (1963) *Statistical Tables for Biological, Agricultural and Medical Research,* 6th edition. Edinburgh: Oliver and Boyd.

Fraser, G. R. & Friedmann, A. I. (1967) *The Causes of Blindness in Childhood.* Baltimore: Johns Hopkins.

Fraser, G. R. & Mayo, O. (1974) Genetical load in man. *Humangenetik,* **23,** 83–110.

Freidhoff, L. B. & Chase, G. (1975) A computer-oriented linkage analysis scheme. *Clin. Genet.,* **7,** 219–26.

Fritze, D., Herrman, C., Naeim, F., Smith, G. S. & Walford, R. I.. (1974) HL-A antigens in myasthenia gravis. *Lancet, i,* 240–2.

Gaines, R. E. & Elston, R. C. (1969) On the probability that a twin pair is monozygotic. *Amer. J. Hum. Genet.,* **21,** 457–65.

Gardner, R. J. M. (1976) Chondrodysplastic short-limbed dwarfism. (In press.)

Gardner-Medwin, D. (1970) Mutation rate in Duchenne type of muscular dystrophy. *J. Med. Genet.,* **7,** 334–7.

Glass, B., Sacks, M. S., Jahn, E. F. & Hess, C. (1952) Genetic drift in a religious isolate: an analysis of the causes of variation in blood group and other gene frequencies in a small population. *Amer. Naturalist,* **86,** 145–59.

Gottesman, I. I. & Shields, J. (1972) *Schizophrenia and Genetics: A Twin Study Vantage Point.* New York: Academic Press.

Gottesman, I. I. & Shields, J. (1973) Genetic theorizing and schizophrenia. *Brit. J. Psychiat.,* **122,** 15–30.

Greenwood, M. & Yule, G. U. (1914) On the determination of size of family and of the distribution of characters in order of birth. *J. Statist. Soc.,* **77,** 179–97.

Haldane, J. B. S. (1938) The estimation of the frequencies of recessive conditions in man. *Ann. Eugen. (Lond.),* **8,** 255–62.

Haldane, J. B. S. & Smith, C. A. B. (1947) A simple exact test for birth-order effect. *Ann. Eugen. (Lond.),* **14,** 117–24.

Hardy, G. H. (1908) Mendelian proportions in a mixed population. *Science,* **28,** 49–50.

Heuch, I. & Li, F. H. F. (1972) PEDIG—A computer programme for calculation of genotype probabilities using phenotype information. *Clin. Genet.,* **3,** 501–4.

Hewitt, D., Milner, J., Csima, A. & Pakula, A. (1971) On Edwards' criterion of seasonality and a non-parametric alternative. *Brit. J. Prev. Soc. Med.,* **25,** 174–6.

Hogben, L. (1931) The genetic analysis of familial traits. I. Single gene substitutions. *J. Genet.,* **25,** 97–112.

Hogben, L. (1946) *An Introduction to Mathematical Genetics.* New York: W. W. Norton Inc.

Holzinger, K. J. (1929) The relative effect of nature and nurture influences on twin differences. *J. Educ. Psychol.,* **20,** 241–8.

Jacob, A., Clack, E. R. & Emery, A. E. H. (1968) Genetic study of sample of 70 patients with myasthenia gravis. *J. Med. Genet.,* **5,** 257–61.

James, W. H. (1972) Secular changes in dizygotic twinning rates. *J. Biosoc. Sci.,* **4,** 427–34.

Johnston, F. E., Jantz, R. L., Kensinger, K. M., Walker, G. F., Allen, F. H. & Walker,

M. E. (1968) Red cell blood groups of the Peruvian Cashinahua. *Hum. Biol.* **40**, 508–16.

Johnston, F. E., Kensinger, K. M., Jantz, R. L. & Walker, G. F. (1969) The population structure of the Peruvian Cashinahua: demographic, genetic and cultural inter-relationships. *Hum. Biol.,* **41**, 29–41.

Jones, K. L., Smith, D. W., Harvey, M. A. S., Hall, B. D. & Quan, L. (1975) Older paternal age and fresh gene mutation: data on additional disorders. *J. Pediat.,* **86**, 84–8.

Kellermann, G., Luyten-Kellermann, M. & Shaw, C. R. (1973) Genetic variation of aryl hydrocarbon hydroxylase in human lymphocytes. *Amer. J. Hum. Genet.,* **25**, 327–31.

Kelly, T. E., Chase, G. A., Kaback, M. M., Kumor, K. & McKusick, V. A. (1975) Tay-Sachs disease: high gene frequency in a non-Jewish population. *Amer. J. Hum. Genet.,* **27**, 287–91.

Kimura, M. and Crow, J. F. (1963) The measurement of effective population number. *Evolution,* **17**, 279–88.

Knudson, A. G., Wayne, L. & Hallett, W. Y. (1967) On the selective advantage of cystic fibrosis heterozygotes. *Amer. J. Hum. Genet.,* **19**, 388–92.

Kosambi, D. D. (1944) The estimation of map distances from recombination values. *Ann. Eugen. (Lond.),* **12**, 172–5.

Kudo, A. & Sakaguchi, K. (1963) A method for calculating the inbreeding coefficient. II. Sex-linked genes. *Amer. J. Hum. Genet.,* **15**, 476–80.

Laberge, C. (1966) Prospectus for genetic studies in the French Canadians with preliminary data on blood groups and consanguinity. *Bull. Johns Hopkins Hosp.,* **118**, 52–68.

Lenz, W. (1961) Kindliche Missbildungen nach Medikament—Einnahme während der Gravidität? *Dtsch. Med. Wschr.,* **86**, 2555–6.

Levitan, M. & Montagu, A. (1971) *Textbook of Human Genetics,* 467. London: Oxford University Press.

Li, C. C. (1961) *Human Genetics.* New York: McGraw-Hill.

Li, C. C. & Mantel, N. (1968) A simple method of estimating the segregation ratio under complete ascertainment. *Amer. J. Hum. Genet.,* **20**, 61–81.

McBride, W. G. (1961) Thalidomide and congenital abnormalities. *Lancet, ii,* 1358.

McDevitt, H. O. & Bodmer, W. F. (1974) HL-A, immune-response genes, and disease. *Lancet, i,* 1269–75.

McKeown, T. & Record, R. G. (1956) Maternal age and birth order as indices of environmental influence. *Amer. J. Hum. Genet.,* **8**, 8–23.

Mayo, O. (1970) On the maintenance of polymorphisms having an inviable homozygote. *Ann. Hum. Genet. (Lond.),* **33**, 307–17.

Morton, N. E. (1959) Genetic tests under incomplete ascertainment. *Amer. J. Hum. Genet.,* **11**, 1–16.

Morton, N. E. & Chung, C. S. (1959) Formal genetics of muscular dystrophy. *Amer. J. Hum. Genet.,* **11**, 360–79.

Mourant, A. E., Kopeć, A. C. & Domaniewska-Sobczak, K. (1958) *The ABO Blood Groups—Comprehensive Tables and Maps of World Distribution.* Oxford: Blackwell.

Murdoch, J. L., Walker, B. A., Hall, J. G., Abbey, H., Smith, K. K. & McKusick, V. A. (1970) Achondroplasia—a genetic and statistical survey. *Ann. Hum. Genet. (Lond.),* **33**, 227–44.

Murdoch, J. L., Walker, B. A. & McKusick, V. A. (1972) Parental age effects on the occurrence of new mutations for the Marfan syndrome. *Ann. Hum. Genet. (Lond.),* **35**, 331–6.

Murphy, E. A. & Chase, G. A. (1975). *Principles of Genetic Counseling.* Chicago: Year Book Medical Publishers.

Murphy, E. A. & Mutalik, G. S. (1969) The application of Bayesian methods in genetic counselling. *Hum. Hered.,* **19,** 126–51.
Myrianthopoulos, N. C. & Aronson, S. M. (1966) Population dynamics of Tay-Sachs disease. I. Reproductive fitness and selection. *Amer. J. Hum. Genet.,* **18,** 313–27.

Neel, J. V. & Schull, W. J. (1954) *Human Heredity.* Chicago: University of Chicago Press.
Nielsen, J. (1967) Inheritance in monozygotic twins. *Lancet, ii,* 717–8.
Nielsen, J., Holm, V. & Haahr, J. (1975) Prevalence of Edwards' syndrome. Clustering and seasonal variation? *Humangenetik,* **26,** 113–16.

Oakes, M. W. (1968) Heterozygous advantage and its relationship to increased heterozygote fertility. *Ann. Hum. Genet. (Lond.),* **32,** 173–81.
Osborne, R. H. & De George, F. V. (1959) *Genetic Basis of Morphological Variation— An Evaluation and Application of the Twin Study Method.* Cambridge, Mass.: Harvard University Press.
Osborne, R. H., Adlersberg, D., De George, F. V. & Wang, C. (1959) Serum lipids, heredity and environment. *Amer. J. Med.,* **26,** 54–9.

Pearn, J. H. (1973) The gene frequency of acute Werdnig-Hoffmann disease (SMA type I). A total population survey of North-East England. *J. Med. Genet.,* **10,** 260–5.
Penrose, L. S. (1953) The genetical background of common diseases. *Acta Genet.,* **4,** 257–65.
Penrose, L. S. (1957) Parental age in achondroplasia and mongolism. *Amer. J. Hum. Genet.,* **9,** 167–9.

Race, R. R. & Sanger, R. (1975) *Blood Groups in Man,* 6th edition. Oxford: Blackwell.
Reed, T. E. (1959) The definition of relative fitness of individuals with specific genetic traits. *Amer. J. Hum. Genet.,* **11,** 137–55.
Reed, T. E. (1969) Caucasian genes in American Negroes. *Science,* **165,** 762–8.
Registrar General (1975) *Statistical Review of England and Wales for the year 1973, Part 2.* London: H.M.S.O.
Registrar General, Scotland. *Annual Reports for 1969–73, Parts 1 and 2.* Edinburgh: H.M.S.O.
Renwick, J. H. (1969) Progress in mapping human autosomes. *Brit. Med. Bull.,* **25,** 65–73.
Renwick, J. H. (1971) The mapping of human chromosomes. *Ann. Rev. Genet.,* **5,** 81–120.
Roberts, D. F. (Ed.) (1975) *Human Variation and Natural Selection.* London: Taylor & Francis.
Roberts, J. A. F. (1957) Blood groups and susceptibility to disease: a review. *Brit. J. Prev. Soc. Med.,* **11,** 107–25.
Roberts, J. A. F. (1973) *An Introduction to Medical Genetics,* 6th edition. London: Oxford University Press.

Salzano, F. M., Neel, J. V. & Maybury-Lewis, D. (1967) Further studies on the Xavante Indians. I. Demographic data on two additional villages: genetic structure of the tribe. *Amer. J. Hum. Genet.,* **19,** 463–89.
Schlosstein, L., Terasaki, P. I., Bluestone, R. & Pearson, C. M. (1973) High association of an HL-A antigen, W 27, with ankylosing spondylitis. *New Engl. J. Med.,* **288,** 704–6.
Shokeir, M. H. K. (1975) Investigation on Huntington's disease in the Canadian prairies. II. Fecundity and fitness. *Clin. Genet.,* **7,** 349–53.
Skinner, R., Emery, A. E. H., Anderson, A. J. B. & Foxall, C. (1975) The detection of carriers of benign (Becker-type) X-linked muscular dystrophy. *J. Med. Genet.,* **12,** 131–4.

Skinner, R., Smith, C. & Emery, A. E. H. (1974) Linkage between the loci for benign (Becker type) X borne muscular dystrophy and deutan colour blindness. *J. Med. Genet.*, **11**, 317–20.

Smith, C. (1970) Heritability of liability and concordance in monozygous twins. *Ann. Hum. Genet. (Lond.)*, **34**, 85–91.

Smith, C. (1972a) Correlation in liability among relatives and concordance in twins. *Hum. Hered.*, **22**, 97–101.

Smith, C. (1972b) Computer programme to estimate recurrence risks for multifactorial familial disease. *Brit. med. J.*, i, 495–7.

Smith, C. (1974) Concordance in twins: methods and interpretation. *Amer. J. Hum. Genet.*, **26**, 454–66.

Smith, C. A. B. (1968) Linkage scores and corrections in simple two- and three-generation families. *Ann. Hum. Genet. (Lond.)*, **32**, 127–50.

Smith, C. A. B. (1972) Note on the estimation of parental age effects. *Ann. Hum. Genet. (Lond.)*, **35**, 337–42.

Smith, S. M. & Penrose, L. S. (1955) Monozygotic and dizygotic twin diagnosis. *Ann. Hum. Genet. (Lond.)*, **19**, 273–89.

Smith, S. M., Penrose, L. S. & Smith, C. A. B. (1961) *Mathematical Tables for Research Workers in Human Genetics.* London and Edinburgh: J. & A. Churchill.

Snedecor, G. W. & Cochran, W. G. (1967) *Statistical Methods,* 6th edition. Ames, Iowa: Iowa State University Press.

Spuhler, J. N. (1963) The scope for natural selection in man. In *Genetic Selection in Man,* ed. Schull, W. J. 1–111. Ann Arbor: University of Michigan Press.

Spuhler, J. N. (1968) Assortative mating with respect to physical characteristics. *Eugen. Quart.*, **15(2)**, 128–40.

Steinberg, A. G. (1959) Methodology in human genetics. *J. Med. Educat.*, **34**, 315–34.

Stevenson, A. C. & Kerr, C. B. (1967) On the distributions of frequencies of mutation to genes determining harmful traits in man. *Mutation Res.*, **4**, 339–52.

Svejgaard, A., Platz, P., Ryder, L. P., Nielsen, L. S. & Thomsen, M. (1975) HL-A and disease associations—a survey. *Transplant. Rev.*, **22**, 3–43.

Tanaka, K. (1974) A new simplified method for estimating relative fitness in man. *Jap. J. Hum. Genet.*, **19**, 195–202.

Thoday, J. M. (1975) Non-Darwinian 'evolution' and biological progress. *Nature (Lond.)*, **255**, 675–7.

Tünte, W., Becker, P. E. & Knorre, G. (1967) Zur Genetik der Myositis ossificans progressiva. *Humangenetik,* **4**, 320–51.

Vogel, F. (1970) ABO blood groups and disease. *Amer. J. Hum. Genet.*, **22**, 464–75.

Vogel, F. & Helmbold, W. (1972) Blutgruppen—Populationsgenetik und Statistik. In *Humangenetik,* ed. Becker, P. Vol. 1, 129–557. Stuttgart: Georg Thieme Verlag.

Vogel, F. & Rathenberg, R. (1975) Spontaneous mutation in man. In *Recent Advances in Human Genetics,* ed. Harris, H. & Hirschhorn, K. Vol. 5, 223–318. New York & London. Plenum Press.

Wagener, D. K. & Cavalli-Sforza, L. L. (1975) Ethnic variation in genetic disease: possible role of hitchhiking and epistasis. *Amer. J. Hum. Genet.*, **27**, 348–64.

Walter, S. D. & Elwood, J. M. (1975) A test for seasonality of events with a variable population at risk. *Brit. J. Prev. Soc. Med.*, **29**, 18–21.

Weinberg, W. (1901) Beiträge zur Physiologie und Pathologie der Mehrlingsgeburten beim Menschen. *Pflügers Arch. ges. Physiol.*, **88**, 346–430.

Weinberg, W. (1908) Über den Nachweis der Vererbung beim Menschen. *Jahresh. Verein f. vaterl. Naturk. in Württemberg,* **64**, 368–82 (see Stern, C. (1943) The Hardy-Weinberg Law. *Science,* **97**, 137–38).

Wiener, A. S. (1970) Blood groups and disease. *Amer. J. Hum. Genet.*, **22**, 476–83.

Woodward, R. H. & Goldsmith, P. L. (1964) *Mathematical and Statistical Techniques for Industry: Monograph No. 3. Cumulative Sum Techniques.* Edinburgh: Oliver and Boyd.

Woolf, B. (1955) On estimating the relation between blood group and disease. *Ann. Hum. Genet. (Lond.),* **19,** 251–3.

Woolf, L. I., McBean, M. S., Woolf, F. M. & Cahalane, S. F. (1975) Phenylketonuria as a balanced polymorphism: the nature of the heterozygote advantage *Ann. Hum. Genet. (Lond.),* **38,** 461–9.

Workman, P. L., Blumberg, B. S. & Cooper, A. J. (1963) Selection, gene migration and polymorphic stability in a U.S. White and Negro Population. *Amer. J. Hum. Genet.,* **15,** 429–37.

Wright, S. (1922) Coefficients of inbreeding and relationship. *Amer. Nat.,* **56,** 330–8.

Wright, S. (1926) Effects of age of parents on characteristics of the guinea pig. *Amer. Naturalist,* **60,** 552–9.

Wright, S. (1948) On the roles of directed and random changes in gene frequency in the genetics of populations. *Evolution,* **2,** 279–94.

Wright, S. (1950/1) The genetical structure of populations. *Ann. Eugen. (Lond.),* **15,** 323 54.

Wynne-Davies, R. (1970) The genetics of some common congenital malformations. In *Modern Trends in Human Genetics.* Ed. Emery, A. E. H. Vol. 1, 316–38. London: Butterworths.

Zatz, M., Itskan, S. B., Sanger, R., Frota-Pessoa, O., & Saldanha, P. H. (1974) New linkage data for the X-linked types of muscular dystrophy and G6PD variants, colour blindness, and Xg blood groups. *J. Med. Genet.,* **11,** 321–7.

Index

Achondroplasia
  mutation rate, 32
  paternal age effect, 107, 113
Acrocephalosyndactyly (Apert's
    syndrome), paternal age effect, 107,
    113, 118
Albinism, 22
Alkaptonuria, 22
Amish, 38
Anencephaly see CNS malformations
Ankylosing spondylitis
  association HLA-B27, 102
  heritability, 54
  inheritance, 53
  recurrence risks, 105
Apert's syndrome, paternal age effect, 107,
    113, 118
Aryl hydrocarbon hydroxylase, 5
Ascertainment
  complete, 37
  multiple incomplete, 48
  single incomplete, 43
Association see Disease association
Assortative mating, 14–16
Autosomal dominant inheritance, tests for,
    35–6
Autosomal gene frequency
  heterozygote not recognizable, 4–5
  heterozygote recognizable, 5–6
  standard error, 5
Average inbreeding coefficient, 19

Bayes' theorem, 89
  see also Recurrence risks
Becker muscular dystrophy
  fitness, 29, 31
  linkage relationships, 74
  recurrence risks, 94
Bernstein's equation, 23
Birth order, population data
  correlations, 117
  means, 113–14
Birth order effect
  examples, 107–8
  methods of estimation

Birth order effect—*continued*
  choice of controls, 112–3
  Greenwood-Yule method, 115
  Haldane and Smith method, 108–12
  partial correlations, 115–20
  see also Parental age effect
Blood groups
  associations, 98–106
  frequencies, 9–10
  linkage (Lutheran), 65–7
Bonferroni inequality, 103

Cashinahua Indians, 13–14
Centimorgan, 70
Cleft lip $+/-$ cleft palate
  heritability, 54
  recurrence risks, 96
Cline, 22
Club foot (congenital)
  heritability, 54
  recurrence risks, 96
CNS malformations
  cyclical changes in incidence, 127–8
  heritability, 54
  maternal age and birth order effects, 108
  recurrence risks, 96
Coefficients
  average inbreeding, 19
  inbreeding (F), 16
  relationship (R), 20
  selection (s), 24
Complete ascertainment
  a priori method, 37
  maximum likelihood method, 39
  'singles' method, 42
Concordance in twins
  heritability from, 60–2
  pairwise, 84
  proband, 84
Congenital malformations
  inheritance, 51
  recurrence risks, 96
Consanguinity, 16 *et seq.*
Correlation
  between parent-offspring, 14, 59

Variance—*continued*
    interpair in twins, 86
    intrapair in twins, 85

Weinberg's method, for determining
    zygosity, 77–8
Werdnig-Hoffmann disease, 5

Xavante Indians, 14
X-linkage, 49–50
X-linked gene

X-linked gene—*continued*
    frequency, 9
    mating types, 9
    offspring types, 9

'z' score *see* Linkage
'z' transformation, 119
Zygosity, twin, diagnosis, fetal membranes,
    78
    similarity, 78–83
    Weinberg's method, 77–8

Filmset by Typesetting Services Ltd, Glasgow and Edinburgh
Printed by T. & A. Constable Ltd, Edinburgh